The American Health Empire: Power, Profits, and Politics

THE
AMERICAN
HEALTH
EMPIRE:

Power, Profits, and Politics

A HEALTH–PAC BOOK *Prepared by*

Barbara & John Ehrenreich

Random House / *New York*

CONTENTS

PREFACE

If this book can be said to have a single thesis, it is that the American health system is not in business for people's health. Traditionally, liberals have explained that America is not a healthy place to live, in either a medical or a social sense, simply because health and other social services are low priority items in a nation whose resources are committed to military and economic expansion. "If we could only spend all the money we spend in Vietnam on hospitals, housing, schools . . ." goes the refrain.

So we have reasoned. But on looking closer, we began to understand that national priorities are only part of the problem, perhaps the more manageable part. Billions of dollars could be diverted from America's aggressive, defensive, and interplanetary enterprises with no appreciable effect on the quality of health care. For even within the institutions that make up America's health system—hospitals, doctors, medical schools, drug companies, health insurance companies—health care does not take the top priority. Health is no more a priority of the American health industry than safe, cheap, efficient, pollution-free transportation is a priority of the American automobile industry. The victims, then, are not just the poor, the blacks, the Puerto Ricans, who cannot afford to buy what the health industry is selling, but also all the millions of middle-class and working-class people who try to extract health services from the health industry.

This book is the outgrowth of studies and analyses of the health system, particularly the New York City health system, done over the last two years. In many ways, New York's health scene is unique in the nation. The city has more doctors, more hospitals, more medical schools, and, of course, more people than any other American city. And its wealth of health resources are perhaps more clearly welded into a "system" than anywhere else in the country. But what makes New York unique also makes it prophetic. The same tendencies, the ascendancy of private medical "empires," the collapse of municipal hospital systems, the failure of Medicaid, the unionization of hospital workers, and the movements of resistance and change among communities, health workers, and health students which we have observed in New York, are evident now in Boston, Pittsburgh, Chicago, San Francisco, and throughout the country.

The book is a collective product of the staff of the Health Policy Advisory Center (Health-PAC). Health-PAC grew out of a 1967 exposé-analysis of New York City municipal hospital policy by Robb Burlage (*New York City's Municipal Hospitals: A Policy Review,* Institute for Policy Studies, Washington, D.C., 1967). This study created a demand for ongoing, topical analysis of city health politics, and in mid-1968, Robb, then working with Maxine Kenny, set up an office and began to publish a monthly *Health-PAC Bulletin.* Beginning in 1969 the staff began to expand; it now consists of 10 full-time people: Robb Burlage, Leslie Cagan, Vicki Cooper, Barbara Ehrenreich, John Ehrenreich, Oliver Fein, Ruth Glick, Maxine Kenny, Kenneth Kimerling, and Howard Levy. In addition, a number of medical, law, and nursing students have worked with us part-time or full-time for short periods.

Health-PAC's activities, originally confined to research and analysis, have expanded to include direct educational projects, such as seminar series for students and community health activists, and direct technical assistance to the student, worker, and community groups that spearhead the movement for change. We have seen ourselves as part of this growing "health movement," and have defined our primary mission as service to it, providing information and analysis of immediate usefulness to people who are active or might become active in health issues. At the same time, we have seen ourselves as serving the larger movement for radical social change in America, by making health a "case study" in the need for democratic restructuring of American institutions.

Our style of work is informal and cooperative. The products of our research are evaluated by the group and fused into our overall analysis. Thus, this book is the work of the entire group —the full-time staff plus the people who have worked with us as student "interns" or seminar participants.

This book represents an attempt by two of us (Barbara and John Ehrenreich) to put together the results of Health-PAC's thinking and working together. About half of the chapters grew directly out of material originally presented in the Health-PAC Bulletin. We have tried to combine the old and new, with a unifying analysis which is true to the spirit and the content of many long discussions at Health-PAC. Various Health-PACers worked directly on the writing of several of the chapters: Robb Burlage, on medical empires; Maxine Kenny, on mental health centers and the Lincoln Hospital insurgency; Oliver Fein, on national health insurance and on the worker and student insurgencies; Mills Matheson (now a medical student at Stanford), on regional medical programs and comprehensive health planning; and Phil Wolfson (a young doctor and friend of Health-PAC), on regional medical programs.

One person who is not a Health-PAC staff member deserves major credit for the ideas expressed here: Harry Becker, now a Professor of Community Medicine at Albert Einstein College of Medicine. He has been a close friend and an energetic teacher —pointing out the important issues, showing us how to investigate them, and helping us understand the results.

We also wish to express our deep gratitude to Mr. Samuel Rubin. He has provided financial support and personal encouragement, while leaving us completely free to determine our own path and our own conclusions. Without him, there would have been no Health-PAC, and no book.

May, 1970

The American Health Empire: Power, Profits, and Politics

I

INTRODUCTION:

THE SYSTEM BEHIND THE CHAOS

The American health crisis became official in 1969. President Nixon announced it in a special message in July. Liberal academic observers of the health scene, from Harvard's John Knowles to Einstein College of Medicine's Martin Cherkasky, hastened to verify the existence of the crisis. Now the media is rushing in with details and documentation. *Time, Fortune, Business Week,* CBS, and NBC, are on the medical scene, and finding it "chaotic," "archaic," and "unmanageable."

For the great majority of Americans, the "health care crisis" is not a TV show or a presidential address; it is an on-going crisis of survival. Every day three million Americans go out in search of medical care. Some find it; others do not. Some are helped by it; others are not. Another twenty million Americans probably ought to enter the daily search for medical help, but are not healthy enough, rich enough, or enterprising enough to try. The obstacles are enormous. Health care is scarce and expensive to begin with. It is dangerously fragmented, and usually offered in an atmosphere of mystery and unaccountability. For many, it is obtained only at the price of humiliation, dependence, or bodily insult. The stakes are high—health,

life, beauty, sanity—and getting higher all the time. But
the odds of winning are low and getting lower.

For the person in search of medical help, the illness or
possibility of illness which prompted the search is quickly
overshadowed by the difficulties of the medical experience
itself:

*Problem One: Finding a place where the appropriate care is
offered at a reasonable price*

For the poor and for many working-class people, this can
be all but impossible. Not long ago it was commonly believed that sheer distance from doctors or hospitals was a
problem only in rural areas. But today's resident of slums
like Brooklyn's Bedford-Stuyvesant, or Chicago's south
side, is as effectively removed from health services as his
relatives who stayed behind in Mississippi. One region of
Bedford-Stuyvesant contains only one practicing physician for a population of one hundred thousand. Milwaukee
County Hospital, the sole source of medical care for tens
of thousands of poor and working-class people, is sixteen
miles outside the city, an hour and a half bus ride for many.
A few years ago, a social science graduate student was able
to carry out her thesis work on rural health problems in a
densely populated Chicago slum.

After getting to the building or office where medical
care is offered, the next problem which affects both poor
and middle-class people is paying for the care. Except at
a diminishing number of charitable facilities, health care is
not free; it is a commodity which consumers purchase
from providers at unregulated, steadily increasing prices.
Insurance plans like Medicaid, Medicare, and Blue Cross
help soften the blow for many, but many other people are

too rich for Medicaid, too poor for Blue Cross, and too young for Medicare. A total of twenty-four million Americans have no health insurance of any variety. Even for those who are insured, costs remain a major problem: first there is the cost of the insurance itself, then there is the cost of all those services which are not covered by insurance. 102 million Americans have no insurance coverage for visits to the doctor, as opposed to hospital stays. They spend about ten dollars just to see a doctor; more, if laboratory tests or specialists are needed. Otherwise, they wait for an illness to become serious enough to warrant hospitalization. Hardly anyone, of course, has insurance for such everyday needs as dental care or prenatal care.

Supposing that one can afford the cost of the care itself, there remains the problem of paying for the time spent getting it. Working people must plan on losing a full workday for a simple doctor's appointment, whether with a private physician or at a hospital clinic. First, there is a long wait to see the doctor. Middle-class people may enjoy comfortable chairs, magazines, and even coffee, while waiting in their doctor's anteroom, but they wait just the same. As busy private doctors try to squeeze more and more customers into their day, their patients are finding that upwards of an hour's wait is part of the price for a five- or ten-minute face-to-face encounter with a harried physician.

Not all kinds of care are as available, or unavailable, as others. In a city studded with major hospitals the person with multiple bullet wounds or a rare and fatal blood disease stands a far better chance of making a successful medical "connection," than the person with stomach pains, or the parents of a feverish child. Hospitals, at all times, and physicians, after 7:00 P.M. (if they can be located) are geared to handling the dramatic and exotic cases which excite professional interest. The more mundane, or less obviously catastrophic, case can wait—and wait. For psychiatric problems, which are probably the nation's single greatest source of disability, there are almost no outpatient facilities, much less sympathetic attention when one finds them. Those of the mentally ill who venture forth in search of help are usually rewarded with imprisonment in a state institution, except for the few who are able to make the investment required for private psychiatric care. Even for the wealthy, borderline problems, like alcoholism and addiction may as well be lived with—there are vanishingly few facilities of any kind to deal with them.

Problem Two: Finding one's way amidst the many available types of medical care

Most of us know what buildings or other locations are possible sources of medical help. Many of us can even arrange to get to these buildings in a reasonable amount of time. But, having arrived at the right spot, the patient finds that his safari has just begun. He must now chop through the tangled morass of medical specialization. The only system to American health services, the patient discovers, is the system used in preparing the tables of contents of medical textbooks. Everything is arranged according to the various specialties and subspecialties doctors study, not according to the symptoms and problems which patients perceive.

The middle-class patient is relatively lucky. He has a private doctor who can serve as a kind of guide. After an initial examination, which may cost as little as five dollars or as much as fifty dollars, the patient's personal doctor sends him to visit a long list of his specialist colleagues—

a hematologist, allergist, cardiologist, endocrinologist, and maybe a urologist. Each of these examines his organ of interest, collects twenty dollars and up, and passes the patient along to the next specialist in line. If the patient is lucky, his illness will be claimed by one of the specialists fairly early in the process. If he is not so lucky, none of them will claim it, or—worse yet—several of them will. Only the very wealthy patient can afford the expense of visiting and retaining two medical specialists.

The hospital clinic patient wanders about in the same jungle, but without a guide. The hospital may screen him for his ills and point him in the right direction, but, from then on, he's on his own. There's nobody to take overall responsibility for his illness. He can only hope that at some point in time and space, one of the many specialty clinics to which he has been sent (each at the cost of a day off from work) will coincide with his disease of the moment.

Just as exasperating as the fragmentation of medical care is the fragmentation of medical care financing. Seymour Thaler, a New York state senator from Queens, likes to tell the story of one of his constituents who came to Thaler's office, pulled out his wallet, and emptied out a stack of cards. "Here's my Medicaid card, my Medicare card, my Blue Cross supplementary card, my workmen's compensation card, and my union retirement health plan card." "So what are you complaining about?" Thaler asked. "I've got a stomach ache," the old man answered, "so what do I do?"

A family makes matters even more complicated and confusing. Grandparents have Medicare, children have Medicaid, the parents may have one or several union hospitalization insurance plans. No one is covered for everything, and no mother is sure just who is covered for what.

If three members of the family came down with the same illness, they would more than likely end up seeing three different doctors, paying for it in three (or more) different ways, and staying in separate hospitals. In 1968, a New York father of six quit his job and applied for welfare, claiming he couldn't work and see to his children's health care. One child, diagnosed as retarded, had to be taken to and from a special school each day. All required dental care, which was free at a Health Department clinic on Manhattan's lower east side. For dental surgery, however, they went to a clinic a bus ride away, at Bellevue. The youngest children went to a neighborhood pediatrician who accepted Medicaid patients. An older child, with a rare metabolic defect, required weekly visits to a private hospital clinic a half hour's trip uptown. The father himself, the victim of a chronic back problem, qualified for care at a union health center on the west side. For him, family health maintenance was a full-time job, not, as it is for most parents, just a busy sideline.

Doctors like to tell us that fragmentation is the price of quality. We should be happy to be seeing a specialist, twice as happy to be seeing two of them, and fully gratified to have everyone in the family seeing a special one of his own. In many difficult cases, specialization does pay off. But evidence is accumulating that care which is targeted at a particular organ often completely misses the mark. Take the case of the Cleveland woman who had both a neurological disease and a damaged kidney. Since the neurologist had no time to chat, and since she assumed that doctors know a good deal more than their patients, she never mentioned her kidney to her neurologist. Over a period of time, her urologist noted a steady deterioration of her kidney problem. Only after the kidney had been removed did the urologist discover that his colleague, the neurologist, had been prescribing a drug which is known to put an extra strain on the kidney.

The patient may have only one problem—as far as his doctors are concerned—and still succumb to medical fragmentation. Recently, an elderly man with a heart condition was discharged from a prestigious private medical center, assured he was good for another decade or two. Four weeks later he died of heart failure. Cause? Overexertion. He lived on the fifth floor of a walk-up apartment—a detail which was obviously out of the purview of his team of hospital physicians, for all the time and technology they had brought to bear on his heart. Until human physiology adapts itself to the fragmentation of modern medical practice, it is up to the patient himself to integrate his medical problems, and to integrate them with the rest of his life.

Problem Three: Figuring out what they are doing to you

Many people are not satisfied to have found the correct doctor or clinic. They also want to know what is being done to their bodies, and why. For most, this is not just idle curiosity. If the patient has to pay all or some of the bill, he wants to know whether a cheaper treatment would be just as efficacious, or whether he should really be paying for something much fancier. The doctors' magazine *Medical Economics* tells the story of the family whose infant developed bronchopneumonia. The physician who visited the home judged from the furnishings that the family could not afford hospitalization. With little or no explanation, he prescribed an antibiotic and left. The baby died six hours later. The parents were enraged when they learned the diagnosis and realized that hospitalization might have helped. They wanted to know the risks, and make the decision themselves.

More commonly, the patients fear they will be over-treated, hence overbilled, for a medical problem. A twenty-five-year-old graduate student, a victim of hayfever, was told by an allergist at prestigious New York Hospital that his case would require several years of multiple, weekly, antiallergy injections. When he asked to know the probability that this treatment would actually cure his hayfever, the allergist told him, "I'm the doctor, not you, and if you don't want to trust my judgment you can find another doctor—or be sick forever for all I care!" Following this advice, the patient did, indeed, find a new doctor. And when the limitations of the treatment were explained to him, he decided the treatment was probably worth the trouble after all. The important thing is that <i>he</i> decided.

Some people, perhaps more trusting of doctors, never ask for an explanation until they have to in sheer self-defense. Residents of Manhattan's lower east side tell the story of the woman who was admitted to a ward at Bellevue for a stomach operation. The operation was scheduled for Thursday. On Wednesday a nurse told her she was to be operated on that day. The patient asked why the change. "Never mind," said the nurse, "give me your glasses." The patient could not see why she should give up her glasses, but finally handed them over at the nurse's insistence. Inside the operating room, the patient was surprised when she was not given general anesthesia. Although her English was poor, she noticed that the doctors were talking about eye cancer, and looking at her eyes. She sat up and said there was nothing wrong with her eyes—her stomach was the problem. She was pushed back on the operating table. With the strength of panic, she leapt up and ran into the hall. A security guard caught her, running sobbing down the hall in an operating gown. She was summarily placed in the psychiatric ward for a week's observation.

Even when confronted with what seems to be irrational therapy, most patients feel helpless to question or complain. A new folklore of medicine has emerged, rivaling that of the old witch doctors. Medical technology, from all that the patient has read in the newspapers, is as complex and mystifying as space technology. Physicians, from all he has seen on TV serials or heard thirdhand from other patients, are steely-nerved, omniscient, medical astronauts. The patient himself is usually sick-feeling, often undressed, a nameless observer in a process which he can never hope to understand. He has been schooled by all the news of medical "space shots"—heart transplants, renal dialysis, wonder drugs, nuclear therapy, etc.—to expect some small miracle in his own case—a magical new prescription drug or an operation. And miracles, by their very nature, are not explainable or understandable. Whether it's a "miracle detergent," a "miracle mouth wash," or a "miracle medical treatment," the customer can only pay the price and hope the product works.

Problem Four: Getting a hearing if things don't go right

Everything about the American medical system seems calculated to maintain the childlike, dependent, and depersonalized condition of the patient. It is bad enough that modern medical technology has been infused by its practitioners with all the mystery and unaccountability of primitive shamanism. What is worse is that the patient is given absolutely no means of judging what care he should get or evaluating what he has gotten. As one Washington, D.C. taxi driver put it, "When I buy a used car, I know it might be a gyp. But I go over it, test it, try to figure out if it's O.K. for the price. Then take last year when I got started getting some stomach problem. The doctor says I need an operation. How do I know I need an operation? But what can I do—I have an operation. Later I get the bill—$1700—and Blue Cross left over $850 for me to pay. How should I know whether the operation should cost $50 or $1700? Now I think my stomach problem is coming back. Do I get my money back?"

Doctors and hospitals have turned patients into "consumers," but patients have none of the rights or protections which consumers of other goods and services expect. People in search of medical care cannot very easily do comparative shopping. When they're sick, they take help wherever they can get it. Besides, patients who switch doctors more than once are viewed by other doctors as possible neurotics. Health consumers know what they'd like—good health—but they have no way of knowing what this should entail in terms of services—a new diet, a prescription, or a thousand-dollar operation. Once they've received the service, the doctor, not their own perception, tells them whether it did any good. And if they suspect that the price was unduly high, the treatment unnecessarily complicated or drastic, there is no one to turn to—no Better Business Bureau or Department of Consumer Protection.

When something goes really wrong—a person is killed or maimed in the course of medical treatment—there is still no formal avenue of recourse for the patient or his survivors. Middle-class people, who know the ropes and have some money to spend, can embark on a long and costly malpractice suit, and win, at best, a cash compensation for the damage done. But this process, like everything else in a person's encounter with doctors and hospitals, is highly individualistic, and has no pay-off in terms of the general health and safety of the community. For the poor, there is usually no resource at all short of open resistance. A Manhattan man, infuriated by his wife's treatment in the emergency room of New York's Beth Israel Medical Center, beat up the intern on duty. Another man, whose child died inexplicably at a big city public hospital, solitarily pickets City Hall summer after summer.

Problem Five: Overcoming the built-in racism and male chauvinism of doctors and hospitals

In the ways that it irritates, exhausts, and occasionally injures patients, the American medical system is not egalitarian. Everything that is bad about American medicine is especially so for Americans who are not male or white. Blacks, and in some areas Indians, Puerto Ricans, or Mexicans, face unique problems of access to medical care, and not just because they are poor. Many hospitals in the south are still unofficially segregated, or at least highly selective. For instance, in towns outside of Orangeburg, South Carolina, blacks claim they are admitted to the hospital only on the recommendation of a (white) employer or other white "reference."

In the big cities of the north, health facilities are available on a more equal footing to blacks, browns, and poor whites. But for the nonwhite patient, the medical experience is more likely to be something he will not look forward to repeating. The first thing he notices about the large hospital—he is more likely to be at a hospital clinic than at a private doctor's office—is that the doctors are almost uniformly white; the nonskilled workers are almost entirely brown or black. Thus the nonwhite patient enters the hospital at the bottom end of its social scale, quite aside from any personal racial prejudices the staff may harbor. And, in medicine, these prejudices take a particularly insulting form. Black and Puerto Rican patients complain again and again of literally being "treated like animals" by everyone from the clerks to the M.D.'s. Since blacks are assumed to be less sensitive than white patients, they get less privacy. Since blacks are assumed to be more ignorant than whites, they get less by way of explanation of what is happening to them. And since they are assumed to be irresponsible and forgetful, they are more likely to be given a drastic, one-shot treatment, instead of a prolonged regimen of drugs, or a restricted diet.

Only a part of this medical racism is due to the racist attitudes of individual medical personnel. The rest is "institutional racism," a built-in feature of the way medicine is learned and practiced in the United States. As interns and residents, young doctors get their training by practicing on the hospital ward and clinic patients—generally nonwhite. Later they make their money by practicing for a paying clientele—generally white. White patients are "customers"; black patients are "teaching material." White patients pay for care with their money; black patients pay with their dignity and their comfort. Clinic patients at the hospital affiliated with Columbia University's medical school recently learned this distinction in a particularly painful way. They had complained that anesthesia was never available in the dental clinic. Finally, a leak from one of the dental interns showed that this was an official policy: the patient's pain is a good guide to the dentist-in-training—it teaches him not to drill too deep. Anesthesia would deaden the pain and dull the intern's learning experience.

Hospitals' institutional racism clearly serves the needs of the medical system, but it is also an instrument of the racist, repressive impulses of the society at large. Black community organizations in New York have charged hospitals with "genocidal" policies towards the black community. Harlem residents tell of medical atrocities—cases where patients have unwittingly given their lives or their organs in the cause of medical research. A more common charge is that, to public hospital doctors, "the birth control method of choice for black women is the hysterectomy." Even some doctors admit that hysterectomies are often performed with pretty slim justification in ghetto hospitals. (After all, they can't be expected to take a pill every day, can they? And one less black baby is one less baby on welfare, isn't it?) If deaths from sloppy abortions run highest in the ghetto, it is partly because black women are afraid to go to the hospital for an abortion or for treatment following a sloppy abortion, fearing that an involuntary sterilization—all for "medical" reasons—will be the likely result. Aside from their medical policies, ghetto hospitals have a reputation as racist because they serve as police strongholds in the community. In the emergency room, cops often outnumber doctors. They interrogate the wounded—often before the doctor does, and pick up any vagrants, police brutality victims, drunks or addicts who have mistakenly come in for help. In fact, during the 1964 riots in New York, the police used Harlem Hospital as a launching pad for their pacification measures.

Women are the other major group of Americans singled out for special treatment by the medical system. Just as blacks face a medical hierarchy dominated by whites, women entering a hospital or doctor's office encounter a hierarchy headed by men, with women as nurses and aides playing subservient, hand-maid roles. And in the medical system, women face all the male supremacist attitudes and superstitions that characterize American society in general —they are the victims of sexism, as blacks are of racism. Women are assumed to be incapable of understanding complex technological explanations, so they are not given any. Women are assumed to be emotional and "difficult," so they are often classified as neurotic well before physical illness has been ruled out. (Note how many tranquilizer ads in medical journals depict women, rather than men, as likely customers.) And women are assumed to be vain, so they are the special prey of the paramedical dieting, cosmetics, and plastic surgery businesses.

Everyone who enters the medical system in search of care quickly finds himself transformed into an object, a mass of organs and pathology. Women have a special handicap—they start out as "objects." Physicians, despite their supposed objectivity and clinical impersonality, share all the sexual hangups of other American men. The sick person who enters the gynecology clinic is the same sex as the sexual "object" who sells cars in the magazine ads. What makes matters worse is that a high proportion of routine medical care for women centers on the most superstitious and fantasy-ridden aspect of female physiology—the reproductive system. Women of all classes almost uniformly hate or fear their gynecologists. The gynecologist plays a controlling role in that aspect of their lives society values most, the sexual aspect—and he knows it. Middle-class women find a man who is either patronizingly jolly, or cold and condescending. Poorer women, using clinics, are more likely to encounter outright brutality and sadism. Of course, black women have it worst of all. A shy teenager from a New York ghetto reports going to the clinic for her first prenatal check-up, and being used as teaching material for an entire class of young, male medical students learning to give pelvic examinations.

Doctors and hospitals treat pregnancy and childbirth, which are probably among the healthier things that women experience, as diseases—to be supervised by doctors and confined to hospitals. Women in other economically advanced countries, such as Holland, receive their prenatal care at home, from nurses, and, if all goes well, are delivered at home by trained midwives. (The Netherlands rank third lowest in infant mortality rate; the U.S. ranks fourteenth!) But for American women, pregnancy and childbirth are just another harrowing, expensive medical procedure. The doctor does it; the woman is essentially passive. Even in large cities, women often have to go from one obstetrician to another before they find one who approves of natural childbirth. Otherwise, childbirth is handled as if it were a surgical operation, even to the point of "scheduling" the event to suit the obstetrician's convenience through the use of possibly dangerous labor-inducing drugs.

Most people who have set out to look for medical care eventually have to conclude that there *is* no American medical system—at least there is no systematic way in America of getting medical help when you need it, without being financially ruined, humiliated, or injured in the process. What system there is—the three hundred thousand doctors, seven thousand hospitals and supporting insurance plans—was clearly not designed to deal with the sick. In fact the one thing you need most in order to qualify for care financially and to survive the process of obtaining it is *health*, plus, of course, a good deal of cunning and resourcefulness. The trouble is that it's almost impossible to stay healthy and strong enough to be able to tackle the medical system. Preventive health care (regular check-ups, chest X-rays, pap tests, etc.) is not a specialty or even an interest of the American medical system.

The price of this double bind—having to be healthy just to stay healthy—is not just consumer frustration and discomfort. The price is lives. The United States ranks fourteenth among the nations of the world in infant mortality, which means that approximately 33,000 American babies under one year old die unnecessarily every year. (Our infant mortality statistics are not, as often asserted, so high because they are "spoiled" by the death rates for blacks. The statistics for white America alone compare unfavorably to those for countries such as Sweden, the Netherlands, Norway, etc.) Mothers also stand a better chance of dying in the United States, where the maternal mortality rate ranks twelfth among the world's nations. The average American man lives five years less than the Swedish man, and his life expectancy is shorter than for males in seventeen other nations. Many American men never live out their already relatively short lifetime, since the chance of dying between ages forty and fifty is twice as high for an American as it is for a Scandinavian. What is perhaps most alarming about these statistics is that they are, in a relative sense, getting worse. The statistics improve a little each year, but at a rate far slower than that for other advanced countries. Gradually, the United States is slipping behind most of the European nations, and even some non-European nations, in its ability to keep its citizens alive.

*   *   *

These are the symptoms: unhealthy statistics, soaring costs and mounting consumer frustration over the quality and even the quantity of medical care. Practically everyone but the A.M.A. agrees that something is drastically wrong. The roster of public figures actively concerned about the health care crisis is beginning to read like *Who's Who in America:* Labor leaders Walter Reuther of the Auto Workers and Harold Gibbons of the Teamsters, businessmen like General James Gavin of Arthur D. Little, Inc., politicians like New York's Mayor John Lindsay and Cleveland's Mayor Carl Stokes, doctors like Michael DeBakey of Baylor College of Medicine, and civil rights leaders like Mrs. Martin Luther King, Jr. and Whitney Young, Jr. With the help of eminent medical economists like Harvard's Rashi Fein and Princeton's Ann Somers, these liberal leaders have come up with a common diagnosis of the problem: the medical care system is in a state of near-chaos. There is no one to blame—medical care is simply adrift, with the winds rising in all directions. In the words of the official pamphlet of the Committee for National Health Insurance (a coalition of one hundred well-known liberals): "The fact is that we do not have a health care system at all. We have a 'nonsystem.'" According to this diagnosis, the health care industry is, in the words of the January, 1970, *Fortune* magazine, a "cottage industry." It is dominated by small, inefficient and uncoordinated enterprises (private doctors, small hospitals, and nursing homes), which add up to a fragmented and wasteful whole —a nonsystem.

Proponents of the nonsystem theory trace the problem to the fact that health care, as a commodity, does not obey the orderly, businesslike laws of economics. With a commodity like bacon, demand reflects people's desire to eat

bacon and ability to pay for bacon. Since the supply grace-
fully adjusts itself to demand, things never get out of hand
—there is a *system* of bacon production and sales. No such
invisible hand of economic law operates in the health market. First, people buy medical care when they have to, not
when they want to or can afford to. Then, when he does
go to purchase care, the consumer is not the one who
decides what and how much to buy—the doctor or hospital
does. In other words, in the medical market place, it is the
supplier who controls the demand. Finally, medical care
suppliers have none of the usual economic incentives to
lower their prices or rationalize their services. Most hospitals receive a large part of their income on a cost-plus basis
from insurance organizations, and couldn't care less about
cost or efficiency. Doctors do not compete on the basis of
price. In fact, given the shortage of doctors (which is maintained by the doctors themselves through the A.M.A.'s
prevention of medical school expansion), they don't have
to compete at all.

Solutions offered by the liberal viewers of the medical
nonsystem are all along the lines of putting the health
industry on a more "rational," i.e., businesslike basis. First,
the consumer should not have to fish in his pocket each
time the need for care arises; he should have some sort of
all-purpose medical credit card. With some form of Na-
tonal Health Insurance, all consumers, rich or poor, would
have the same amount of medical credit, paid for by the
government, by the consumer, or both through payroll
taxes (see chapter XII). Second, the delivery of health services must be made more efficient. Just as supermarkets
are more efficient than corner groceries, and shopping
centers are more efficient than isolated supermarkets, the

medical system ought to be more efficient if it were bigger and more integrated at all levels. Doctors should be encouraged to come together into group practices, and group practices, hospitals and medical schools should be gradually knitted together into coordinated regional medical care systems. Since they are the centers of medical technology, the medical schools should be the centers and leaders of these regional systems—regulating quality in the "outposts," training professional and paraprofessional personnel, and planning to meet changing needs(see chapters II-VI).

There is only one thing wrong with this analysis of the health care crisis: it's based on a false assumption. The medical reformers have assumed, understandably enough, that the function of the American health industry is to provide adequate health care to the American people. From this it is easy enough to conclude that there is no American health *system*. But this is like assuming that the function of the TV networks is to give comprehensive, penetrating, and meaningful information to the viewers— a premise which would quickly lead us to believe that the networks have fallen into wild disorganization and confusion. Like the mass media, the American medical industry has many items on its agenda other than service to the consumers. Analyzed in terms of all of its functions, the medical industry emerges as a coherent, highly organized system. One particular function—patient care—may be getting slighted, and there may be some problems in other areas as well, but it remains a *system*, and can only be analyzed as such.

The most obvious function of the American medical system, other than patient care, is profit-making. When it comes to making money, the health industry is an extraordinarily well-organized and efficient machine. The most profitable small business around is the private practice of medicine, with aggregate profits running into the billions. The most profitable big business in America is the manufacture and sale of drugs. Rivaling the drug industry for Wall Street attention is the burgeoning hospital supply and equipment industry, with products ranging from chicken soup to catheters and heart-lung machines. The fledgling nursing home (for profit) industry was a speculator's dream in 1968 and 1969, and even the stolid insurance companies gross over ten billion dollars a year in health insurance premiums. In fact, the health business is so profitable that even the "nonprofit" hospitals make profits. All that "nonprofit" means is that the hospital's profit, i.e., the difference between its income and its expenditures, is not distributed to shareholders. These nonprofits are used to finance the expansion of medical empires—to buy real estate, stocks, plush new buildings, and expensively salaried professional employees. The medical system may not be doing too well at fighting disease, but, as any broker will testify, it's one of the healthiest businesses around.

Next in the medical system's list of priorities is research. Again, if this undertaking is measured in terms of its dividends for patient care, it comes out looking pretty unsystematic and disorganized. Although the vast federal appropriations for biomedical research are primarily motivated by the hope of improving health care, only a small fraction (much smaller than need be) of the work done in the name of medical research leaks out to the general public as improved medical care. But medical research has a *raison d'être* wholly independent of the delivery of health services, as an indispensable part of the nation's giant research and development enterprise. Since the Second World War, the United States has developed a vast machinery for R.&D. in all areas—physics, electronics, aerospace as well as biomedical sciences—financed largely by the government and carried out in universities and private industry. It has generated military and aerospace technology, and all the many little innovations which fuel the expansion of private industry.

For the purposes of this growing R.&D. effort, the medical system is important because it happens to be the place where R.&D. in general comes into contact with human material. Medical research is the link. The nation's major biomedical research institutes are affiliated to hospitals to a significant extent because they require human material to carry out their own, usually abstract, investigations. For instance, a sophisticated (and possible patentable) technique for investigating protein structure was recently developed through the use of the blood of several dozen victims of a rare and fatal bone marrow disease. Even the research carried out inside hospitals has implications for the entire R.&D. enterprise. Investigations of the pulmonary disorders of patients in Harlem Hospital may provide insights for designing space suits, or it may contribute to the technology of aerosol dissemination of nerve gas. Or, of course, it may simply lead to yet another investigation.

Human bodies are not all that the medical care system offers up to R.&D. The sociological and psychological research carried out in hospitals and ghetto health centers may have pay-offs in the form of new counterinsurgency techniques for use at home and abroad. And who knows what sinister—or benignly academic—ends are met by the routine neurological and drug research carried out on the nation's millions of mental hospital inmates?

Finally, an important function of the medical care system is the reproduction of its key personnel—physicians. Here, again, there seems to be no system if patient care is the ultimate goal. The medical schools graduate each year just a few more doctors than are needed to replace the ones who retire, and far too few doctors to keep up with the growth of population. Of those who graduate, a growing proportion go straight into academic government, or industrial biomedical research, and never see a patient. The rest, according to some dissatisfied medical students, aren't trained to take care of patients anyway—having been educated chiefly in academic medicine (a mixture of basic sciences and "interesting" pathology). But all this is not as irrational as it seems. The limited size of medical school classes has been maintained through the diligent, and entirely systematic, efforts of the A.M.A. Too many—or even enough—doctors would mean lower profits for those already in practice. And the research orientation of medical education simply reflects the medical schools' own consuming preoccupation with research.

Profits, research and teaching, then, are independent functions of the medical system, not just adjuncts to patient care. But they do not go on along separate tracks, removed from patient care. Patients are the indispensable ingredient of medical profit-making, research, and education. In order that the medical industry serve these functions, patient care must be twisted to meet the needs of these other "medical" enterprises.

Different groups of patients serve the ends of profit-making, research and education in different ways. The rich, of course, do much to keep medical care profitable. They can afford luxury, so, for them, the medical system produces a luxury commodity—the most painstaking, supertechnological treatment possible; special cosmetic care to preserve youth, or to add or subtract fatty tissue; even sumptuous private hospital rooms with carpeting and a selection of wines at meals. The poor, on the other hand, serve chiefly to subsidize medical research and education —with their bodies. City and county hospitals and the wards and clinics of private hospitals provide free care for the poor, who, in turn, provide their bodies for young doctors to practice on and for researchers to experiment with. The lucky poor patient with a rare or interesting disease may qualify for someone's research project, and end up receiving the technically most advanced care. But most of the poor are no more interesting than they are profitable, and receive minimal, low-quality care from bored young interns.

The majority of Americans have enough money to buy their way out of being used for research, but not enough to buy luxury care. Medical care for the middle class is, like any other commodity, aimed at a mass market: the profits are based on volume, not on high quality. The rich man may have his steak dinners catered to him individually; the middle-class consumer waits for his hamburger in the check-out line at the A&P. Similarly, the middle-class patient waits in crowded waiting rooms, receives five minutes of brusque, impersonal attention from a doctor who is quicker to farm him out to a specialist than to take the time to treat him himself, and finally is charged all that the market will bear. Preventive care is out of the question: it is neither very profitable nor interesting to the modern, science-oriented M.D.

The crisis experienced by the poor and middle-class consumer of health care can be traced directly to the fact that patient care is not the only, or even the primary, aim

of the medical care system. But what has turned the consumer's private nightmare into a great public debate about
the health care crisis is that the other functions of the
system are also in trouble. Profit-making, research, and
education are all increasingly suffering from financial
shortage on the one hand and institutional inadequacies on
the other. The solutions offered by the growing chorus of
medical reformers are, in large measure, aimed at salvag-
ing profits, research, and education as much as they are
aimed at improving patient care. They are simple survival
measures, aimed at preserving and strengthening the
medical system as it now operates.

No one, so far, has seen through the proposed reforms.
Union and management groups, who have moved into the
forefront of the medical reform movement, seem happy to
go along with the prescription that the medical system is
writing for itself. The alternative—to marshall all the force
of public power to take medical care out of the arena of
private enterprise and recreate it as a public system, a
community service, is rarely mentioned, and never considered seriously. To do this would be to challenge some of
the underlying tenets of the American free enterprise system. If physicians were to become community employees,
if the drug companies were to be nationalized—then why
not expropriate the oil and coal industries, or the automobile industry? There is an even more direct antipathy to
nationalizing the health industry: a host of industries, including the aerospace industry, the electronic industry,
the chemical industry, and the insurance industry, all have
a direct stake in the profitability of the medical care system. (And a much larger sector of American industry
stands to profit from the human technology spun off by the
medical research enterprise.) Of course, the argument

never takes this form. Both business and unions assert, in their public pronouncements, that only a private enterprise system is capable of managing medical services in an efficient, nonbureaucratic, and flexible manner. (The obvious extrapolation, that all medical services, including voluntary and city hospitals, would be in better shape if run as profit-making enterprises, is already being advanced by a few of the more visionary medical reformers.)

For all these reasons, business and unions (and, as a result, government) are not interested in restructuring the medical care system in ways contrary to those already put forth by the doctors, hospitals, and medical industry companies. Their only remaining choice is to go along with the reforms which have been proposed, in the hope that lower costs, and possibly even more effective care, will somehow fall out as by-products.

For the health care consumer, this is a slim hope. What he is up against now, what he will be up against even after the best-intentioned reform measures, is a system in which health care is itself only a by-product, secondary to the priorities of profits, research, and training. The danger is that, when all the current reforms are said and done, the system as a whole will be tighter, more efficient, and harder to crack, while health services, from the consumer's point of view, will be no less chaotic and inadequate. Health care will remain a commodity, to be purchased at great effort and expense, and not a right to be freely exercised.

But there are already the beginnings of a consumer rebellion against the reformer-managers of the medical care system (see chapter XVI). The demand is to turn the medical system upside down, putting human care on top, placing research and education at its service, and putting profit-making aside. Ultimately, the growing movement of health care consumers does not want to "consume" health care at all, on any terms. They want to take it—because they have to have it—even if this means creating a wholly new American health care system.

II

FROM FAMILY DOCTOR

TO MEDICAL-INDUSTRIAL COMPLEX:

HOW THE SYSTEM GREW

The proper study of the American health system is no longer medicine but medical institutions. Everyone knows that, except in A.M.A. inspirational literature, the myth of the paternal, house-calling practitioner went out years ago. But people are only beginning to discern the outlines of the new medical establishment, based in local networks of hospitals and medical schools, backed up by a highly technological and profitable health commodities industry, and represented nationally by the corporate voices of the American Hospital Association, Blue Cross and the American Association of Medical Schools. At the heart of the new system is no longer the free enterprise private practitioner, but the local, medical-school-centered medical empire. Socially justified by their "scientific" approach to medical care and their "nonprofit" organizational status, the empires provide the perfect front for the nonpatient care missions of the medical research establishment and the medical commodities industries. Closely linked to local nonmedical power structures, the empires provide a firm political footing for the new national medical establishment—Blue Cross, the A.H.A., etc.

The pre-World War II health care system was built around the solo practitioner. The sick person received a physician's services; in return he paid the physician, out of his own pocket, for each service rendered. More than half of the nation's total expenditures for personal health care went for such one-to-one transactions with doctors, dentists, and other practitioners. By present standards, the prewar hospital was a primitive institution offering little more than hotel services for the sick, a few assistants for the doctor, and a certain amount of equipment unavailable in the doctor's private office.

The medical power structure of the prewar period could be summed up in one magic set of letters—the A.M.A. The American Medical Association was the voice of the nation's physicians. Doctors were spread throughout the country, and since they tended to be the wealthier men of their communities, they could exert great political pressure on America's rural-dominated political system. In matters of medical politics, the A.M.A. reigned supreme. The crowning point of its political achievements was the defeat of health insurance measures proposed along with the 1935 Social Security Act, and its repeat performance in laying to rest the postwar national health insurance proposals.

The postwar period has seen a steep decline in the role of the solo practitioner, both in the delivery of medical care itself, and in the medical power structure. Just as at the turn of the century the small factory gave way to the vast corporation, so the tens of thousands of one-man medical entrepreneurs have ceded the field to medical institutions —hospitals, and medical schools. In 1969, less than twenty-nine percent of the nation's health expenditures went to private practitioners of all types; thirty-eight percent went to hospitals alone, and more than sixty percent went to all the panoply of institutionalized health services, from hospital and nursing homes to public health agencies and institutional-based health education and research.

The shift of the center of medical gravity is the result of three complementary forces: changes in technology, changes in financing, and changes in the prestige structure of the medical profession. First, medical care has become vastly more specialized and more dependent on technology. As a result of the last twenty years' technological advances, the old general practitioner, who would listen to grandad's cough, check baby's rash, and perhaps offer a little family counseling all in one home visit, is vanishing along with memories of gramophones and Model T Fords.

But the price paid by the doctors for today's medical-scientific expertise has been a large measure of their independence. A specialist can no more practice in isolation than his organ specialty (eyes, chest, gut, etc.) can function in isolation. With the expanding technology of patient care, doctors find that more and more of their private patients require the personnel and equipment resources of a hospital. No doctor could hope to stock his own office with all the expensive new tools of his trade, or hope to employ a full team of nurses, lab technicians, X-ray technicians, inhalation therapists, and other highly skilled helpers. Then the more specialized the physician, the more he needs the company or proximity of other specialists. Those in his own field help him keep on top of the latest advances in treatment technology, while specialists in other fields supply him, through referrals, with new patients. The result is that today only fifty percent of the nation's physicians are in solo practice, compared to seventy percent in 1950. The rest practice in hospitals, group practices or other health institutions. The doctor's office has been displaced from the center to the periphery of modern medical care; and the doctor himself has become a vassal to what was once just a rent-free workshop—the hospital.

Technology made hospitals important to doctors. But it was the growth of health insurance plans which made hospitals independently viable institutions, with a potential for growth. Essentially all of the means of financing health services which flourished in the postwar period— Blue Cross, commercial health insurance, Medicare, the federal Hill-Burton program for hospital construction— have been oriented toward financing hospitals, not doctors. With the growth of the hospital insurance plans, hospitals could depend on a guaranteed income, and did not have to rely on the state of the patient's bank account at the particular time of the patient's illness. Better yet, most of the hospital insurance plans pay the hospitals on a cost-plus basis, so that hospitals feel free to expand or buy new equipment, knowing that the costs, almost *any* costs, will automatically be covered.

Far from being jealous of the hospitals' financial stability, doctors have actually fought against insurance schemes to cover their own costs. Fearing that outside financing would lead to outside control of medical practice, the doctors saw health insurance as a threat to their independence. But the widespread use of hospital insurance, as opposed to insurance for doctors' care, has ended up making the doctor still more dependent on the hospital. When extensive diagnostic work is required, the doctor knows his patient can't afford to get it on an outpatient basis. So he has the patient admitted to a hospital where the work will be done, and Blue Cross, or some other insurance plan, will pay the bill.

Many doctors begrudge the hospitals their growing dominance, seeing institutionalized medicine as a threat to the hallowed doctor-patient relationship. But a whole new breed of doctors, spawned by the hospitals and medical schools, is growing up with no other home than the large teaching hospital and its labs. In the last two decades the federal government has poured billions of dollars into biomedical research, to the point where research has become the central activity of the country's major medical schools. Many a student groomed in these new research-teaching centers would rather have a longshot crack at the Nobel prize than make $100,000 a year comforting wealthy patients. But the only place you can do research is in a large university-based medical school center: that's where the grants are, the equipment, and the colleagues who make research fun and productive. In the eyes of the new scientist-physician, the old solo practice office is a throwback to a pretechnological era. Hospitals and medical schools are the source of all that's new and the home of all the "really good" physicians.

No sooner had the hospital replaced the doctor as the center of modern medicine, than a third phase of development began. Just as doctors had become dependent on hospitals, individual hospitals were becoming dependent on the medical schools and major teaching hospitals. Community hospitals found they couldn't attract the best young interns and residents, or older private doctors, unless they had some sort of an affiliation with a medical school or major teaching hospital. City and county hospitals found they could hardly attract any interns and residents without prestigious affiliations. In New York City, almost all the hospitals and health centers have come under the medical guidance, through affiliation arrangements made in the last two decades, of one or another of the city's seven medical schools. In Baltimore, Johns Hopkins Medical College, and in Boston, Harvard, are the great medical centers from which affiliations radiate out to the nearby hospitals. The resulting medical empires—networks of affiliated institutions—have replaced the individual hospital as the basic units of modern medicine, just as surely as the hospitals have replaced the private doctors' offices (for more about empires, see chapters III-VI).

The centralization of the health care delivery system around major teaching centers testifies to the growing importance of research and teaching as priorities of the health care system. But the prestige-giving affiliations which have linked hospitals into medical empires dominated by medical schools are not simply marriages of convenience. Major medical institutions are beginning to display an internal dynamic of their own, compelling them to expand through more and more affiliations, more and more new buildings. Profits are not the motivation since, at least for tax purposes, major medical institutions are nonprofit corporations. Medical empires grow because they have to, just in order to maintain their status and prestige. To attract top professors, top physicians and top researchers requires having something to offer them. And something to offer them means other people like themselves, spacious facilities, the latest equipment, and plenty of patients to use as research and teaching material. Affiliated hospitals supply the patients for research material; plentiful federal research grants pay for the illustrious personnel and the fancy equipment. Of course, it takes a research reputation to win the affiliations, and it takes a topflight staff to win the research grants. Even community service programs, such as neighborhood health and mental health centers, are founts of heavy federal funding and a new source of patients for research and teaching. As more and more medical empires take form, the competition for grants and men gets stiffer, and expansion becomes more frenetic. In every major city, medical empires are growing for growth's sake—sweeping up hospitals, health centers, doctors and patients.

Imperial expansion begets power, and power aids the growth of the empire. Control over local health resources leads inevitably to a controlling voice in the politics of local and national health policy. Wherever local decisions about hospital planning and financing are made, as on the boards of directors of Blue Cross and hospital planning agencies, the representatives of local medical empires can be found in force, outnumbering and outweighing the representatives of small, independent hospitals and county medical societies (local units of the A.M.A.). Influence in these private governments, Blue Cross, and the planning agencies, is increasingly matched by imperial influence in local and national public health policy. Imperial representatives can be found in city hall or in Washington, serving as consultants, as members of official commissions, or even as public officials themselves.

Unlike the A.M.A. or its local chapters, which have sought positions of public influence largely for defensive reasons, the medical empires have positive, expansionary reasons for their civic activities. The more hospitals, health centers, nursing homes, etc., that an empire controls, the broader its concern with health policy issues. And, of course, the greater its political role, the more likely it is to acquire new hospitals, health centers, nursing homes, etc.

The medical empires have not, however, simply boot-strapped themselves into their present position of size and authority. For a variety of reasons, forces outside the major hospitals and medical schools have promoted and abetted imperial growth. Blue Cross and other hospital financing agencies find empires attractive on economic grounds. To a Blue Cross plan which covers an entire metropolitan region, it's far less costly to concentrate expensive equipment and facilities in one central medical institution than to duplicate them in each of several smaller institutions. Not only is duplication itself expensive, but it's inefficient to place expensive new equipment in institutions which are not already rich in technological resources and know-how. Thus Blue Cross, acting alone or through local quasi-official hospital planning agencies, has encouraged the centralization of medical technological resources, in a few major institutions—leaving smaller institutions to affiliate with the larger, or be left outside the mainstream of medical technology. The rich get richer, and the poor get more dependent.

The heavy equipment which has come to play such a determining role in the shape of local health service delivery systems is, of course, as profitable to sell as it is expensive to buy (see chapter VII). The companies which manufacture and build hospital computers, hyperbaric chambers, defibrillators, and the like, represent a new outside force which takes a kindly view of the growth of medical empires. Solo doctors do not buy seventy-thousand-dollar cobalt units, or even thirty-thousand-dollar scintillation counters; neither do small community hospitals. Major medical centers are the *only* market for many of the products of the fast-growing hospital equipment industry. Medical empires themselves, as networks of health facilities, are the only market for many of the products now being developed for future sales, such as computers and electronic communications devices designed to link all the electronic equipment in all of an empire's separate facilities. The more that medical technology is packaged and marketed for imperial use, the more necessary and seemingly rational it becomes that empires should dominate local health systems.

But it was the federal government, perhaps more than any other nonmedical force, which promoted the 1960s' consolidation of the health system. The Eighty-eighth and Eighty-ninth Congresses rang with the rhetoric of equality and quality of medical care for all, and produced a spate of legislation which seemed to add up to a whole "Health New Deal." With Medicaid and Medicare, the government underwrote the health costs of millions of former charity patients, providing the financial fuel for the expanding medical empires, and, less directly, for the growing hospital equipment industry (see chapter XI). Having become a major hospital financier, the government, like Blue Cross, became concerned with rationalizing the health delivery system. With one hand, the government was pouring out billions for biomedical research; with the other hand, it was now pouring out billions for patient care. But the research expenditures seemed to have little impact on the quality or costs of patient care. The problem, then, from the federal government's point of view, was to restructure the delivery system so that it would be an efficient outlet for the fruits of the new medical technology. In this undertaking, the Kennedy-Johnson administrations turned to the major medical centers, rather than to the medical professional organizations. The empires had the technology, the medical systems-analysis skills, and a liberal outlook more in line with Kennedy-Johnson politics than that of the right-leaning A.M.A. Thus the federal health system reorganizational programs, like Regional Medical Programs (see chapter XV) and Comprehensive Health Planning (see chapter XIV), were designed to be little more than invitations to the empires to take a larger responsibility in the planning and design of local health systems.

With the sixties' Health New Deal, the empires moved into a position of national eminence. "Regional medical complexes," i.e., medical empires, became the reorganizational dream of federal health planning technicians and policy-makers alike. Prominent medical imperialists, deans of medical schools, directors of major teaching hospitals, etc., began to play a larger role at congressional hearings on presidential commissions, and in the politics of H.E.W. A new national health establishment was emerging and the A.M.A. was no longer all that a congressman needed to know about health politics. A whole roster of national organizations representing institutionalized medicine were beginning to exert their weight: the American Hospital Association, national Blue Cross, and the American Association of Medical Colleges.

The medical empires which rose to dominance in the 1960s are the building blocks of the new health system of the 1970s. The new system is highly organized, institutionalized, and centralized, with major interlocks to health financing institutions, government, and the health commodities and equipment industry. It is, in short, a system. If sometimes it appears disorganized and unsystematic, it is because remnants of the old doctor-centered system still hang on and overlap with the new. The A.M.A., based in the remaining tens of thousands of small city solo practitioners, is alive and well enough to kick up quite a fuss from time to time. In 1964, it threw all its weight against Medicare, managed to win some major concessions, but lost the battle all the same. In 1969, the A.M.A. remarshalled its forces and blocked the appointment of liberal, medical-empire-based, Dr. John Knowles, to a high H.E.W. post. But, having shot its bolt on that fight, the A.M.A. succumbed without a word to the appointment of the equally liberal, empire-oriented Dr. Roger Egeberg to the same post. Now the A.M.A., conceding the growing dependence of its members on hospitals, is throwing its energies into an epic battle with the American Hospital Association—demanding greater power for physicians within the hospitals.

The battles go on, but the war is over. The percentage of physicians who are A.M.A members has dropped eight points in the last ten years, and the A.M.A.'s public credibility has dropped even faster. While the A.M.A. pours its money into symbolic battles and public relations face-lifting, the empires are steadily, confidently, building. There is no going back for the American health system any more than there is for American industry in general. The age of the guild-dominated, individual medical craftsman is over.

III

NEW YORK: THE EMPIRE CITY

"Where should we picket? Who's responsible?" asks the mother, whose daughter, hit by a car, has been kept waiting for hours in the hospital emergency room, after waiting for an hour in the street for the ambulance to come. "Is it the hospital administrator, the mayor, the medical society, or who?"

The answer, in most major American cities, is becoming less and less mysterious. Increasingly, control of health resources and facilities has become centralized in a few towering medical-school-linked systems. In most cities one or two medical centers, such as Johns Hopkins in Baltimore, or the University of Southern California Medical Center in Los Angeles, monopolize local health services. New York City, which has more hospitals, more doctors, and more health dollars per consumer (and more consumers per square foot) than any other American city, is dominated by seven of these medical empires, which together control more than three-quarters of the city's hospital beds, more than half of its health professional resources, and the lion's share of public money for biomedical and sociomedical research and development. In the city's ghetto and lower working-class neighborhoods the imperial sway is near absolute. At least two million New Yorkers are wholly dependent, and another four million partially dependent, on these medical empires for their health and strength.

The medical empires are under private, elite control, but their authority is rooted in law, and their power is rooted in public tax money. For instance, New York City's empires in their present form were forged in the early sixties, when the local municipal hospital department invited medical schools and major voluntary hospitals to affiliate, for a generous subsidy, with the city's twenty-one city-run (municipal) hospitals. Under this program (which has been imitated in cities across the country) the city provided the buildings, the money and the paramedical staff; the medical centers provided professional staff and policy leadership. One by one, the affiliation contracts knitted the municipal hospitals into medical networks under the hegemony of the medical schools and the city's sectarian, philanthropic interest groups.

The affiliation program gave the city's leading private institutions day-to-day control over the operation of the city's half-billion dollar per year public hospital system. But even before the affiliation program, these institutions had an iron grip on the planning and financing of the city's public and private health facilities. Through the state-sanctioned, but private, Health and Hospital Planning Council (see chapter XIV), the empires held final authority over the construction and renovation of all health facilities in the southern New York region. This Council operates as a private club for the medical empires, philanthropic organizations, and Blue Cross, a place where imperial plans are exchanged, conflicts resolved, and turf divided. Through the state-sanctioned, but private, Blue Cross plan, the empires' representatives, along with their counterparts from the world of private industry, decide whom shall be in-

sured for what services and, of course, how much each
hospital shall be paid for its services. (see chapter X). In
other cities as well as New York, medical empires have
found Blue Cross boards of directors and health planning
councils to be congenial instruments for the exercise of
imperial power over a wide range of social issues.

The empires' prestige and wealth is ultimately vested in
their unchallenged monopoly of public funds for health
science education and research. In New York City, more
than several hundred million dollars a year is allocated for
medical research alone, largely through federal research
grants. When local control of the Regional Medical Program (see chapter XV) was given to the Associated Medical Schools of Greater New York, the gift was more of a
tribute to imperial power over research and education,
than an extension of it.

As imperial control over public hospitals, planning, and
research and education grows, almost every form of public
funding of health becomes a subsidy to the empires. Medicaid funds in New York City have gone largely to private,
empire-related hospitals (see chapter XI). Since the mid-
sixties, as government funds have created neighborhood
health centers, community mental health centers, and
other "out-reach" programs, these facilities have followed
the public hospitals into the "trusteeship" of one or the
other of the city's medical empires. More recently, a bond
issue in New York State will provide public funds for
construction to go directly to private hospitals, with no
strings attached. And, through the 1969-70 creation of a
quasi-public corporation to manage the city's municipal
hospitals, imperial control over the public hospital expenditures will tighten, and become less open to public
scrutiny.

Imperial power has not simply accrued, step by step, with the flow of public funds to the medical centers. Underlying the empires' growth is an internal dynamic which leads to outward expansion, usually into ghetto areas, and to concentration of brains, facilities, money, and power at the center's core. As teaching and research programs have expanded, these institutions have sought greater access to "teaching material" (poor patients), through control of outposts such as public hospitals and neighborhood health centers. At the same time, the expansion of core activities of research, training, and private patient care, has required central physical expansion—the addition of labs, private pavilions, and housing for faculty and staff.

With philanthropic support dwindling, the empires have had to rely on public support for growth in both dimensions. Public support, in turn, must be wooed with impressive demonstrations of research prowess, "social commitment" or both. More recently, with Viet-nam bleeding research and education budgets, there has been a growing need to consolidate administrative power internally, to try to achieve economies of scale through heightened internal integration around the medical school or private hospital imperial center.

These medical empires and their organizational fronts, such as the Health and Hospital Planning Council, are viewed as the nearest thing to regional governments of health in New York City. One of the key questions in the city is health politics thus becomes: Who controls them and toward what ends? Six of the city's medical school centers are private, as are their major hospital centers. The seventh is state-controlled. All are ultimately controlled by elite boards of trustees representing narrow commercial and corporate interests, including real estate, banking, construction, insurance, and drug and hospital supply interests which profit directly from their hospital association. Sharing imperial trusteeship are the sectarian philanthropic organizations representing the city's traditional ethnic political forces, once power-based in ward- and parish-level charitable activities.

Trustees shape the overall contour of their empires, controlling long range planning, and determining their institutions' choice of banks, construction firms, and real estate agents. Internal medical policy and management—whom shall be served, at what cost and by what means—falls primarily to the medical staff and administration. These groups are divided into two broad factions, both of which lack a comprehensive, accountable public service commitment.

The *patricians*, primarily found among the basic clinical faculties and funded particularly through the National Institutes of Health and private foundations in categorical biomedical research programs, style themselves as the elite defenders of scientific medicine. They are frequently so caught up in their own narrow projects and subspecialties that they resent any intrusions of social reality or broad professional responsibility. These, they say, are social problems for the practitioners (to whom they see themselves relating as teachers and scientific explorers) public health administrators, and politicians—so long as the patricians themselves are reserved an important high priest role to conserve quality. In New York City, this faction is best represented by the medical directorship of the Columbia University College of Physicians and Surgeons.

The *promoters*, on the other hand, based primarily

among the deans, administrators, grantsmen, planners, and more socially oriented medical faculty, are more inclined to invoke the "social medicine" responsibilities of the major medical centers. They prize general H.E.W. funds, as well as local government and privately funded service-oriented grants, for general community and administrative medicine programs and demonstration projects. And in return for large public and private grants, they frequently promise programmatic results they are not really capable of delivering. They are often outspoken in their demands for more rational and modernized organization of medical education, finances, planning, and services delivery—with their own vested definitions and myths about how to solve them. But they usually have remained insulated from, or arrogantly unresponsive to, the needs of their powerless constituents. Almost all have nothing but contempt for government and public accountability, which they consider to be nothing but second-rate administration and red tape. Throughout the nation, there is probably no greater stronghold of medical promotership than the directorship of the Einstein-Montefiore medical empire in New York City (described in chapter V).

The turn to the university-affiliated medical empires to handle the public's medical bags has happened because of the twin failures of local governmental health management and of private medical professional responsibility. For example in 1960, most of New York's municipal hospitals, because of red tape and long-standing fiscal and administrative neglect, didn't seem able to revamp their physical plants and programs to meet the overwhelming demand, particularly for emergency and walk-in medical services, and to recruit American-trained house staffs and the best-trained attending staffs. At that time there was not sufficient consumer organization and public demand to restructure the pattern of city government management of health services. Nor were the private, medical-society-related physicians who volunteered care in the municipal hospitals able to rise to the task of providing leadership for reorganization. Thus the affiliation plan was created quickly and loosely to get some new private professional resources into the municipal hospitals from the private medical schools and voluntary hospitals. To many of the private empire promoters, the affiliation plan was seen as only the first step toward a total private takeover of the municipal hospitals.

A new medical myth emerged to defend the salience of these private institutions as the elite guardians of the public's health. Because of their wide-ranging geographical influence, the empires were supposedly capable of providing regional integration and cooperation of health facilities. Because of their research and teaching expertise, they were seen as able to provide high quality care in the municipal hospitals. And, because of their internal, baronial management systems, they were looked to to provide managerial flexibility for the municipal hospitals. Contrasted to the antisocial fragmentation of care perpetrated by the city's solo practioners, and to the present inflexibility and low quality of most public institutions, the appeal of such relatively benevolent autocracies was strong.

But the private, university-connected empires have failed to deliver in all areas of promised performance. Regionalization around a center of medical excellence has been practiced only insofar as it benefits the empire's center, never its outposts. In New York City's empires, regionalization has meant little more than top-down administrative control of health facilities, and has meant nothing in terms of integration and coordination for the patients' convenience. The asserted ability of the major teaching hospitals to provide quality care has been apparent only for certain specialized and "interesting" treatment and diagnostic procedures. The empires' control has usually been antagonistic to the achievement of medical quality in social terms, i.e., comprehensive, low-cost, patient-centered services. Finally, managerial flexibility in some of the city's medical empires has bordered on criminal abandon. As revealed in 1968 state investigations of the New York City affiliation program, public funds for patient care in city hospitals have been shuffled and redealt at imperial whim, often vanishing into private research enterprises, doubled salaries for private staff members, equipment destined for the imperial core, and even parties and travel bonuses for imperial staff serving in municipal hospitals.

Malfeasance by the private empires charged with administering public funds and facilities would be a serious enough breach of public trust. But, in many cases, the narrow research, teaching, and profit priorities of the private empires have actually led to worsened conditions in the public hospitals, greater fragmentation, dehumanization, and neglect of basic health services. Through the affiliation program, medical empires gained greater power of selection over their patient intake, dumping uninteresting and nonpaying patients on their affiliated public hospitals. In turn, the empire-controlled affiliation staffs at the city hospitals are also more interested in maintaining an interesting mix of patients than in providing public health services, and they dump the least interesting patients on to the city's dumps of last resort—Bellevue, Kings County, Harlem Hospital, etc. If the patient dies in transit while being dumped—as scores are known to have done—that is not considered the fault of the institution which rejected him. In municipal hospitals affiliated with private empires, patients have undergone dangerous and unnecessary diagnostic procedures, chemotherapy and surgery, not in the interests of treatment, but in the interests of research. Finally, each of the city's medical empires has become a center of bulldozing real estate expansion, mowing down neighborhoods and dislocating community facilities, without any comprehensive physical plan and certainly without any community involvement in shaping this form of "urban redevelopment."

Imperial malfeasance has provoked exposés, outcries, and increasingly, insurgencies. But empires are still on the upswing, expanding to claim more and more public programs, contracting to escape community protests, and engulfing more and more of the city's medical manpower and funding resources. Faced with the scientific rationality of the empires, A.M.A. style doctor power has withered to a pathetic, rearguard status, or retreated to the suburbs. Faced with the empires' oversold managerial know-how, the local public health agencies have eclipsed themselves to the role of obedient check signers, handing over public tax money for an increasingly private health enterprise.

But this increasing monopolization of urban medical power carries the seeds of its own destruction. People no longer face an anonymous and diffuse local health system whose authority is scattered between public agencies, professional organizations, philanthropies, and health institutions. More and more neighborhoods, in more and more cities, face a single, clearly identifiable, medical empire. As these empires become more top-heavy, more centralized and more dependent on public money, they become more vulnerable—easier to identify and hold responsible.

IV

COLUMBIA: THE RELUCTANT EMPIRE

There are rumbles in the Columbia (College of Physicians and Surgeons) medical empire that some observers think may be heard around the world. On the downtown Columbia campus (at 116th Street—the medical campus is "uptown," at Columbia-Presbyterian Medical Center, west of 168th Street and Broadway), notorious for its gymnasium and defense contracts and the 1968 campus siege, general faculty and students now talk about the vulnerability of Columbia "medical gymnasiums" uptown. They fear that these might at any moment get Columbia into even more momentous warfare with the Harlem and Washington Heights communities.

What is this medical Columbia all about? It is a medical teaching, research, and service complex concentrated in the Washington Heights-Harlem-Upper West Side area of Manhattan. Built around Columbia-Presbyterian Medical Center, the largest voluntary hospital center in New York City; it also includes two other major voluntary teaching hospitals, St. Luke's and Roosevelt; and two municipal hospitals with which it is affiliated—Harlem Hospital Center and Francis Delafield; and it has intimate ties with scores of other medical institutions in the New York area. The entire Columbia medical complex includes more than 4,500 hospital beds, counting more than 1,540 at Pres-

byterian and 885 at Harlem City Hospital Center, and
involves the annual training in the hospitals of about 750
interns and residents.

The Columbia-Presbyterian Medical Center complex is
far more than a medical center in the narrow sense. It is
an international professional organization and a vast and
wealthy financial empire, serving and depending on the
support of U.S. business and government. The empire is
an essentially closed corporation. It is one of the richest
medical centers in the world. Total assets were $180 mil-
lion in 1968, and growing at ten percent a year. Presbyterian Hospital alone has an operating income of $53
million and every year but one since 1958 has made a net
gain or profit (this does not include income from investments). Government money, coming through Medicaid,
Medicare, and research grants, now covers more than half
the medical center's bills. Philanthropic contributions account for only 1.2 percent of income. The medical center
has vast real estate holdings in the Washington Heights
area, comparable to the downtown Columbia campus' estate in Morningside Heights and is currently buying up
tenements at the phenomenal rate of $500 worth of prop-
erty per hour.

It has microbiology research contracts with the Army
and the Navy and has research and training outlets in
Beirut, Taipei, Buenos Aires, and on private rubber planta-
tions in Latin America.

Beyond its own immediately affiliated institutions uptown, it has major Brooklyn and Cooperstown hospital
center affiliations and has attached to its faculty the directors of pathology at fifty-two hospitals in the greater New
York area.

The center has as the president of its major teaching

hospital a Texaco director, and has the president of U.S. Steel chairing the finance committee, and the president of A.T.&T. chairing the planning and real estate committee.

It has the presidents of a number of national professional specialty associations and the chairmen of numerous National Institutes of Health project committees on its faculty.

It has a former medical school dean as a department chairman, supplied the new dean of New York Medical College a year ago from its professorial ranks, and just spun off formerly-affiliated Mount Sinai Hospital as a new medical school.

And yet, Columbia is, in some ways, a reluctant empire, particularly with regard to establishing itself as a vast medical service organization in the Harlem-Washington Heights area. Faculty patricians have been highly resistant to medical empire promoters on its own faculty and staff. In December 1968 at Columbia, one of the nation's most prominent aggregators and defenders of academically-based, private medical empires, Dr. Ray E. Trussel, threw in the towel and headed for a major hospital administration post on the lower east side.

Who rules the empire?

Columbia, loosely chaired by Dean H. Houston Merritt, operates as a confederation of departmental baronies held together by research and publishing contracts, and an endless input of graduate student and house staff apprentices whose careers depend on their blessing. Dean Merritt surrounds himself with associates as expediters and deflectors, such as old-liner Dr. George A. Perera (Dean of Students and of Admissions, who recently urged a crackdown on student beards and long hair); the more liberal Dr. Douglas S. Damrosch (although he was the administrator responsible recently for denying Columbia meeting space to employees wishing to discuss a unionization campaign); and research-prestigious Dr. Melvin D. Yahr (a noted neurologist, director of the well-known Parkinson's Disease Clinic, and the dean's emissary to Harlem, known for his effective use of Negro physician liaison figures there).

Columbia-Presbyterian and the other hospitals in the empire balance between the courtier tastes of the medical faculty and the philanthropic, finance, real estate, and special program interests of the trustees. Presbyterian Executive Vice President Alvin J. Binkert is the expediting chief —he even operates (*sans* M.D.) as a powerful member of the Medical Board. Significantly, Merritt and Binkert are cochairmen of the Joint Committee of the Faculty and the Medical Board of the Facilities of the Medical Center and are known empire-wide as the "Joint Committee."

The Trustees of Columbia University, of course, are already celebrated from the 1968 student rebellion as a kind of uptown approximation of the executive committee of the U.S. ruling class, with some Columbia urban renewal and real estate interests thrown in. Columbia-Presbyterian's trustees resemble the University trustees in personal and in social disposition—primarily corporate-financial and Republican. (Trustees of Roosevelt and St. Luke's affiliated hospitals consist more of New York philanthropic and civic types who no doubt take their lead from the "big boards," both financially and medically.)

Despite (or because of) Columbia's power, rising discontent among medical and nursing students, workers, and residents of the Washington Heights community threatens the empire's present state of enterprise: a disparate set of black physician and community forces, prominently centered in Harlem CORE's "Committee of 100," have been calling for community control, not only of Columbia-affiliated Harlem City Hospital but of all health services in the greater Harlem area. Columbia, they charge, has proved itself unwilling to use the medical resources it controls for the benefit of the community, and has jealously excluded the community from participating in the control of these resources. Black physicians for example are angry about being excluded from important positions in the academically controlled Columbia-Presbyterian network and about the difficulties they face in getting their patients admitted to the best services. Harlem people have been deeply frustrated about the slowness in completing the new Harlem Hospital building, which finally opened in 1969 after literally decades of anticipation and a capital budget promise since the late 1950s. "A rock in the ground would grow faster," said one Harlem militant.

Harlem Hospital itself is a major focus of community resentment. Although supported by a generally quite dedicated medical and paramedical staff, the hospital is forced to be a surgery-happy buffer and receiving hospital, overwhelmed by patients dumped on it by surrounding Columbia-affiliated research and teaching-oriented voluntary hospitals, especially Presbyterian. A black physician at Harlem wrote in 1968 that "black physicians and the general community alike are outraged by the numerous cases of literally genocidal medical treatment and patient rejection because of narrow research interests. . . ." A new breed of socially committed young physicians are now being recruited among the Harlem house staff, but it still shows the strains of an assignment where blacks are exiled and where those with a yen to cut are attracted. It is reputed to be one of the best hospitals in the world to be treated for acute trauma, such as gunshot and stab wounds.

But the specialty clinics have waiting lists from three weeks to two months. The pressure of patients hurriedly dumped to Harlem Hospital because of scientific disinterest or socioeconomic aversion was expressed dramatically in the case of one elderly patient who was hustled out of Presbyterian Hospital to Harlem so quickly that the tubing was still hanging loose from an incompleted intravenous procedure.

The opening of the new Harlem Hospital building in 1969 failed to produce the expected mollifying effect. For one thing, due to the long delay in construction, the new building was obsolete before it opened. It features outdated, charity era six-person wards, which are officially ineligible for Medicare and Medicaid reimbursement and illegal under the 1965 State Hospital Code. Provision for desperately needed prenatal, pediatric and obstetrical care is less than adequate. But by the time the building finally opened, distrust of Columbia and disgust with the city bureaucracy ran so deep that it wouldn't have mattered what the building contained. At a town meeting to celebrate the opening, hospital and city officials were assailed by community residents with charges that Harlem Hospital exists solely to provide guinea pigs for Columbia's research.

Many of Harlem's more militant spokesmen feel that, as a matter of community defense, the hospital and all other local health facilities should be spun off from both Columbia and the central city administration, into direct community control. When the bill establishing a public corporation to operate all the city hospitals was passed in the spring of 1969, CORE and some black legislators managed to sneak in an amendment which allowed Harlem Hospital to decentralize immediately from the central corporation. CORE intends to push this legislative foot-in-the-door for all it's worth, despite the city's concerted opposition. Community control would mean, among other things, community control of the more than fifteen million dollars a year (including more than one million a year overhead, or profit) now paid to Columbia for its affiliation with Harlem Hospital.

Given Columbia's performance in Harlem, it is no wonder that Harlem residents were bitter about Columbia; about Dean Houston Merritt rushing to treat Portuguese dictator Salazar for a severe stroke (when most Harlem stroke victims are considered scientifically uninteresting at Presbyterian); about the rise of a new fifteen-story private ambulatory care facility next door to Presbyterian for the private and semiprivate patients of Columbia faculty (while the clinics for the poor at Presbyterian are in notoriously poor condition); about the (ultimately ill-fated) Columbia speculative sponsorship of a new cigarette filter and of its recent receipt of grants for development of advanced organ transplant engineering (when a few more dollars and more attention for prenatal care might save the lives of thousands of infants in Harlem over a period of time). In fact, Columbia's reputation as a major center for the treatment of, for example, heart disease and stroke, makes it all the more anathema to the surrounding community.

There is also community bitterness about the educational walls around Columbia, seemingly insurmountable to blacks and Puerto Ricans. In 1970 there were only about fifteen black and Puerto Rican students in the entire Columbia medical student body of about 450 and, except for the nursing school, there are precious few Columbia paramedical and new-health-careers development programs. (City University and Mount Sinai Medical College plan to establish a four-year health-careers college in East Harlem within the next year or so.) Little effort has been made to recruit students from poor backgrounds or to enrich the Columbia curriculum and educational pattern to become more relevant and accessible to them. Rather than reconsidering the discriminatory socioeconomic narrowness of its student selection—stressed in demands for change being made by current medical student leaders themselves—the Columbia catalog boasts only of the superscientific excellence of its past selections.

Columbia has recently hired a public relations firm to improve its image, especially in the black and Puerto Rican communities. Its Urban Center (Ford Foundation money) has funded a Committee on Health Priorities for Harlem to conduct professional and community workshops to smooth the rough edges. Even so, relationships have deteriorated to such an extent that Columbia has been blocked by the community from buying property for nurses' residences near the site of the new Harlem Hospital.

Workers within Columbia share much of the community's resentment of the empire, plus some grievances of their own. At Presbyterian Hospital, workers found themselves up against the laboratory wall during a recent union organizing drive by Drug and Hospital Workers Local 1199 among medical school employees. The administration of Columbia pulled out all stops against union organizers who approached their technical, service, and clerical staffs. Besides making it difficult for the group to obtain meeting rooms and sabotaging leaflet campaigns, the hospital administration set up an informal spy network made up of "loyal" employees of the medical center "who can be counted on in times of crisis." This counterinsurgency force was described in a captured document (a report to Columbia from a private consulting firm) which included the dossiers which had been compiled on the workers: For example, one pro-union medical school doctor was described by an informant as a rabid civil rights advocate, but according to the document, the informer thought that the doctor might oversell the union and so antagonize people. Another group of workers was singled out for having signed a petition asking for wages comparable to the medical school-affiliated Presbyterian Hospital.

About the last place the Columbia empire expected trouble from was the student body—traditionally a clean-cut corps of graduates from the "best" schools. So it was a total surprise in the spring of 1969 when fifty white-coated Columbia students marched into the Presbyterian clinic waiting rooms and began leafleting the patients about their school's low level of commitment to its own motto, "Better health care for all regardless. . . ." Through a summer-long campaign of petitioning patients, the students picked up a wide range of community support, from the local Reform Democrats to the Black Panther Party. The resulting community, medical, and nursing student coalition demanded that the Presbyterian clinic be run by a community board and that it begin to decentralize to more convenient neighborhood settings. An argument repeated again and again in the coalition's leaflets was that Columbia, despite its reputation as a world leader in health, lagged well behind most other New York medical centers in attention to the ghetto on its doorstep.

Columbia faculty patricians have resisted Columbia's growing involvement with the community, despite mounting student, worker, and community discontent, and despite the community's usefulness as "teaching

material." They blame Dr. Trussell (former Dean of the
School of Public Health and former New York City Hospital Commissioner) and his associates for getting them
into the turbulent environment of Harlem and Washington Heights in the first place.

Dr. Trussell almost single-handedly engineered Columbia's affiliation with Harlem Hospital, bucking considerable opposition from the more isolationist faculty
members. In 1961 when he was City Hospital Commissioner, Trussell almost literally signed the Harlem
Hospital affiliation contract with himself—as City Commissioner and as Director of Columbia's School of Public
Health without the support of the Department of Medicine at Columbia. The Public Health School, at least in the
short run, had to mobilize much of the medical staff for
Harlem, because of the Department of Medicine's initial
veto. For more than six years the faculty cold war went on,
but the Columbia-Harlem Hospital relationship thickened,
while it became obvious that Columbia's days at Bellevue
(where Columbia had been affiliated for years) were num-
bered. In 1967-68, N.Y.U. took full control at Bellevue, and
Columbia moved its Bellevue Division full-time staff and
house staff rotation to Harlem, Presbyterian, etc.

There had been a lot of dissatisfaction at Columbia about
the city's underfinancing of Bellevue and the great distance of the hospital, (which is on the lower east side of
Manhattan,) from Columbia. But, on the other hand, some
of the faculty were loathe to move into darkest Harlem,
which was thought to have the worst hospital physical
plant and the most overwhelming patient population in the
city. Besides, if one starts seeing people at Harlem, who
knows, they might start thinking they can see one at Presbyterian—and then what will it all come to? A wing at

Bellevue seemed manageable; an open door to Harlem
seemed, as Dean Merritt observed, a more "unlimited"
commitment of Columbia resources:

> Although the medical-center concept may be ideal, it is not
> always possible or even desirable to concentrate all the clinical
> facilities of a community in close association with the medical
> school. . . . A problem arises . . . when a medical school is called
> upon to help a voluntary or municipal hospital improve its care
> of patients and training of the intern and resident staff. The
> capabilities of the faculty are not unlimited. Dissipation of
> their energies may impair the efficiency of their teaching and
> their research potential. Each school must examine its con-
> science to determine how far it can go in helping to solve this
> problem.

Internal resistance to integrating Columbia's precious
resources with the surrounding community has in some
cases had direct academic backlash effects. One of the
reasons the School of Dental and Oral Surgery came close
to losing its national accreditation in 1964 was lack of access
to a meaningful scale of patient population. When the
School of Public Health's reputation began to skid in the
early 1960s, it was commented that much of the faculty was
doing consulting work or was active somewhere else in the
nation or world (the School is even providing back-up for
a Latin American Center for Medical Administration in
Buenos Aires, Argentina) and was not spending the time
doing effective teaching and service preceptorship in the
immediate environs.

In the past, the members of dissident groups—students,
workers, and community residents—have waged separate,
narrowly defined battles against Columbia's medical
monolith. But in recent months, the three groups have
been getting together for an all-out offensive. Emphasis has

been on demanding greater community worker control over the flow of public finance to the empire and over the empire's real estate business. Ultimately their demand is that Columbia Medical Center be transformed into a public utility, directly accountable to the Harlem-Washington Heights community and to the larger community of health service consumers. Until then, Harlem is at the mercy of the empire's whim and can, at best, keep hat in hand and pray for a change of heart. And cancer. And stroke.

V

EINSTEIN-MONTEFIORE:

OUTWARD BOUND

The Bronx medical empire of Montefiore Medical Center and Albert Einstein Medical College (of Yeshiva University) is well-known among liberal medical reformers nationally and locally as a kind of benevolent private monopoly of health services for almost 1.5 million people. The Bronx ranges from prosperous and booming in the north to desperately poor and decaying in the south. Once the front line of Jewish out-migration from teeming Manhattan, the Bronx now serves the same function for other minority groups. Half the borough's residents are black or Puerto Rican.

Dr. Martin Cherkasky, for almost two decades medical director at Montefiore, and now also chairman of Einstein's Department of Preventive Medicine and Community Health, is considered the house liberal of the national medical establishment. He often speaks in Washington or is quoted in national magazines in favor of group practice, national health insurance, planning, regulating medical quality, and against the freewheeling fee-for-service style of his conservative profession.

It came as something of a shock, therefore, when numerous professional, political, and community forces chose recently to bite this hand that is supposed to feed them. The first shots were fired in the spring of 1968 when Dr. Cherkasky announced that Einstein-Montefiore was developing a plan for the creation of a unified Bronx authority for health services. His announcement was greeted with some of the expected foundation and government financial support. Significantly, however, it was met also with accusations of "fraud" and "imperialism" from some of the people who have to live with the Einstein-Montefiore medical empire.

In the summer of 1968, angry residents of the Hunts Point section of the south Bronx took over David Susskind's national television show, featuring Dr. Cherkasky, to charge that Montefiore and Einstein were neglecting the needs of their area.

A few months later Citywide Health and Mental Health Council, the association of neighborhood-based health and mental health organizations, gave priority to an organizing program to "fight the monopoly of health and mental health by Albert Einstein." Especially with reference to Lincoln Hospital, it pledged to "back up the fight of Bronx community leaders and workers for control of health and mental health services."

Workers at Einstein's Lincoln Community Mental Health Center (both professional and nonprofessional) joined the rebellion against the empire in the spring of 1969, in what was one of the year's most militant, and least publicized, labor actions (see chapter XVIII). Charging Einstein with "malfeasance, inefficiency, chaos, and racism," they seized the center buildings, threw out the administrators, and began to operate the center under worker, community, and patient control. Einstein finally squashed the rebellion (but not the rebels themselves) with a shrewd blend of threats, manipulation of latent divisions between the black and Puerto Rican workers, and police violence.

Students at Einstein participated in the Student Health Organization's 1969 disruption of the national meeting of medical school deans from the American Association of Medical Colleges in Chicago. They attacked the elitism and racism of major medical schools across the nation, demanding that health services and medical education be controlled by the community. Back at school in the spring of 1969, the entire first-year class walked out on a Cherkasky lecture in the community medicine course, demanding that the course be used as a forum for community spokesmen, not the medical school elite. When the Lincoln Mental Health Center rebellion broke out, a number of Einstein students joined the workers in the occupied center, and led support actions on campus.

House staff at Einstein-affiliated Bronx Municipal Hospital defied administration threats of dismissal in early 1969 by urging clinic patients not to pay their sixteen-dollar-per-visit bills. Joining with their patients to announce that clinic bills would henceforth be sent on by patients to the City Hospital Commissioner, they forced the city to reduce clinic fees throughout the city.

In 1968, Bronx Borough President Herman Badillo announced, "I'm putting Einstein on notice that I'm not approving any demonstration projects until we meet minimal health needs." Badillo declared prophetically, months before the Lincoln Mental Health action, "The next area where community control is going to become an important factor is going to be in health services, and the reason for that is that people in slum areas have been asking for better health care over the years. There has been an inadequate response, and the people are coming to feel that if they have control of the health centers and of the hospitals, that they will be able to provide themselves better health care."

The empire which is now the focus of so much hostility —from Bronx residents, public officials, and even its own students and young professionals—began humbly enough. Montefiore's present site was originally an army camp for Confederate prisoners, where one of the P.O.W.'s set up a prison hospital during his stay. (Lincoln Hospital in the south Bronx, now affiliated with Einstein, was set up before the Civil War as a home for aging escaped slaves.) After the war, the former army camp infirmary was transformed into "Montefiore," a chronic care home, by Sir Moses Montefiore, an English banker and philanthropist. It was rejuvenated and expanded into a general hospital in the 1930s by an energetic director, Dr. E.M. Bluestone. During the 1950s Dr. Martin Cherkasky, as director, launched Montefiore on its present empire-expanding course.

Einstein Medical College, Montefiore's partner in progress, grew out of Yeshiva University's post-World War II plan to promote a new Bronx general city hospital, and then to graft on a medical school with full rights to the hospital's teaching material. As New York City Commissioner of Hospitals in the mid-fifties, Dr. Marcus Kogel engineered the actual development of a 1,400-bed Bronx Municipal Hospital Center. Opening cost of this city grant to the future medical school was forty million dollars for construction of Bronx Municipal Hospital, eight million dollars for a nursing school building, and sixty-three acres of city parkland. Kogel went on from his stint with the city to become the first dean of the newly opened Einstein

College of Medicine. The College opened in 1955, and affiliated with Montefiore in 1961.

Since the mid-1950s, Montefiore has increased its physical development around the original buildings about fourfold, and it now even has the approval of Health and Hospital Planning Council (the agency which passes on all hospital construction plans in the New York area) to move the 400-bed Morrisania City Hospital from a low-income southwest neighborhood to the Montefiore grounds in the middle-class upper northwest. As a result, institutional and professional resources have become increasingly heavily concentrated in the upper part of the Bronx, far from the low-income population concentrated in the south Bronx.

Considered "eminent domain" for Einstein-Montefiore are the two other sizable voluntary hospitals in the Borough, 570-bed Bronx-Lebanon in the west Bronx (also part of the Federation of Jewish Philanthropies) and 330-bed Misericordia in the northeast (a Catholic institution, currently the private affiliating hospital for 400-bed Fordham City Hospital in the west central Bronx). Dr. Cherkasky has physicians whom he considers his own people (part-time faculty in Einstein's Department of Community Health) in key program development spots at these two voluntary hospitals. Various approaches are being made by empire promoters toward a Montefiore merger with Bronx-Lebanon and toward a Misericordia-Fordham affiliation with Einstein-Montefiore.

* * *

Only the narrow Harlem River separates the Einstein-Montefiore empire from the Columbia empire, but in philosophy and operating style the two empires are poles apart. Columbia Presbyterian Medical Center is withdrawn and patrician about its meager inroads into Harlem and Washington Heights. Einstein-Montefiore aggressively promotes a boroughwide framework with itself at the helm. Columbia shrinks from further public involvement through affiliations. Einstein-Montefiore aspires to control the Bronx—hospitals, health centers, and all. Columbia, especially since its cigarette filter adventure and student explosion of the last two years, shyly avoids the press. Einstein-Montefiore employs a full-time P.R. staff plugged into TV, national magazines, and major newspapers.

In short, Einstein-Montefiore does not behave like a traditional medical school-hospital complex. What gives a nonprofit, academically-based organizational complex the profit motif of an Einstein-Montefiore? To most observers, the dynamics of Einstein-Montefiore expansionism are beyond economic law or organizational logic, and Einstein-Montefiore is written off as a case of medical liberalism run wild. Liberalism is part of the answer. The Einstein-Montefiore trusteeship network, centered in the Federation of Jewish Philanthropies, does not exactly correspond with the predominantly WASP banker-financier-internationalist world of the downtown medical school trusteeships.

Liberalism, however, is only the permissive atmosphere in which an Einstein-Montefiore thrives—the motivating force surges out of the inner logic of the new government and philanthropic granting and funding system. Einstein-Montefiore has been riding the cycle of grants and demonstration projects. It sponsors medical demonstrations which advertise for and justify the next grant, hence the next project, and so on. As dependence on public funding has grown, so has Einstein-Montefiore's need for ever greater public trust and appreciation—always wooed with new, more dazzling meaning? The price of this reliance on public support is the continual fear of being upstaged by a yet-unconquered institution, or dethroned by an angry community. Einstein-Montefiore must always be one step ahead of the competition and the public—it must *plan*, erecting vast frameworks of control and defense. Plans, in turn, are themselves marketable to the federal and foundation funding axis, which is increasingly nervous about the chaos of our national medical "nonsystem".

Einstein and Montefiore, both separately and in association, were among the first institutions in the country to make well-packaged "medical progress" their product. They have sold pioneering breakthroughs, demonstrations, and social commitment and gained the reputation for being where the scientific and social action is in medicine. Einstein and Montefiore have underwritten "demonstration projects" as kinds of philanthropic good will and advertising costs—from the Family Health Maintenance Demonstration in the fifties to the Neighborhood Medical Care Demonstration today. This latter project, a typical Einstein-Montefiore effort, is a "continuous, comprehensive, family-oriented" health center in the southwest Bronx, is staffed and controlled by Montefiore Hospital and serves perhaps as many as 10,000 persons now, with 30,000 more projected (perhaps overoptimistically). Neighborhood Medical Care Demonstration (recently renamed the "Martin Luther King Health Center") has been much lauded in many major magazines and has the highest "reporter-patient" ratio in America.

The academic counterpart of the field demonstrations is Dr. Cherkasky's mushrooming Department of Preventive

Medicine and Community Health at Einstein. (The retainer list of "faculty" for this department is a "Who's Hustling" in New York City health politics—from the Borough President's health affairs aide to Dr. Cherkasky's scouts at Misericordia and Bronx-Lebanon Hospitals.)

The human side to the demonstration project proliferation is the in-gathering to the imperial fold of bright, dedicated personnel. Dr. Cherkasky is particularly well-known as a recruiter of potential innovators to do their thing, as long as "their thing" is a grant-lucrative demonstration project, and they are willing to do it through his channels and under his command. This view of progress as an individual project-hustle pervades the Einstein-Montefiore sheltered workshop for social progress, leading even the most socially dedicated people to function in a constricted, elitist style. They learn to accept crushing compromises in their original conceptions because they appear to feel there is nowhere else they could get paid as well to do their thing as well. Despite vetoes and frustrations, the bright young men keep coming, and, as they accumulate, it becomes easier to attract new ones; hence, new project grants; hence more bright young men, etc.

Progress-packaging and personnel-processing are the dynamics of the empire's expansion—the fuel is public money. Like so many other so-called private institutions, Einstein and Montefiore have built their empire on public tax dollars, land, and institutions. The city's initial investment in the empire was the land and funds for the construction of Bronx Municipal Hospital as the teaching hospital for Einstein. The City has continued to pour money into the empire to pay for the imperial affiliations to Bronx city hospitals: $250 million in the last decade, $30 million in the last year. In addition, the empire receives inestimable amounts of public money via Medicaid and Medicare (for patients in Montefiore and Einstein College Hospital), and via federal research grants (about $20 million in 1967 alone).

With such heavy reliance on public resources, Einstein-Montefiore has had to take an increasingly active role in molding opinion and policy determination. Einstein's associate dean served in 1967 as staff director for the Mayoral Commission which was the godfather of the plan for a quasi-public corporation to run the municipal hospitals. Dr. Cherkasky serves on the city tax-supported Health Research Council (which recently awarded Einstein-Montefiore a major grant for boroughwide planning), on the Blue Cross Board of Directors, and on Health and Hospital Planning Council committees. Concerned with popular opinion as well as public policy, Cherkasky maintains a hefty public relations staff to handle and arrange interviews for TV, congressional hearings, and national magazines.

A consequence of Einstein-Montefiore's heavy public funding, especially of the special project variety, is considerable freedom for the administrators from the prestigious and busy lay trustees. The trustees have little to say about the extramural activities funded directly from Washington or out of individual private family or foundation pockets. Many of the research and program grants come through the Montefiore administrator's or the Einstein dean's office as lump sums and are combined in strange financial ways, impenetrable to *post facto* audit. Other grants come in the name of an individual, faculty or staff and are outside the purview of trustees. As one trustee reportedly described his role, "We are sitting on top of a floating crap game and all we can do [being check-signers] is to say yea or nay to the administrator or dean."

Thus, the relationships which individual administrators and staff develop in the system of financial support—from H.E.W. advisory committees and N.I.H. project committees, to foundation, philanthropic, Blue Cross, regional Health and Hospital Planning Council, and state-local government command posts—frequently become the *de facto* base of personal power within the institution. Internally, the Einstein-Montefiore institutions are structured along the now classic lines of postwar biomedical research grant baronies built into particular departments. In addition, at the top levels, general administrators are able to do their own empire building on a massive scale outside the control of the lay trustees. At all levels, institutional leaders are essentially accountable to nothing but their own professional honor—even for that extra electron microscope stored in a crate in the basement, or for those subspecialty clinics they've organized to match their research needs, rather than the needs and convenience of the community. Unaccountable to and unfettered by lay or public supervision, the Einstein-Montefiore departmental and institutional leaders have become the avant garde of the new class of biomedical and sociomedical entrepreneurs.

*   *   *

Having accumulated such vast resources and power, the empire builders have found it in their interest to begin rationalizing and consolidating the empire. One reason for rationalization is to lower the empire's overhead costs and maximize its funding base. An overriding objective is to carry out preemptive organizational reform (at least in rhetorical terms): (1) to prevent the development of any serious movement for a broadly accountable, truly public health system for the Bronx, and (2) to prevent the emergence of insurgent community and health-worker forces demanding control over the health services on which they so urgently depend.

The consolidation and rationalization effort is itself a kind of demonstration project, with special grants (from New York City's Health Research Council, the Rockefeller Foundation, and others), and burgeoning special staffs. The market for the Bronx plan and similar efforts is the national corporate managers and local power structure leaders. In their growing concern about ghetto rebellions, urban fiscal crises, and uncontrollable costs of medical care, they are turning to the more activist and prestigious wing of medicine (exemplified by Einstein-Montefiore) to cure our sick medical system. Another source of encouragement for these rationalizing efforts is the growth of the health hardware and systems industries. Aircraft companies such as North American, conglomerates such as Litton Industries, and consulting firms, such as Einstein-Lincoln Hospital's contractual management consultant, U.S.R.&D. Corporation, are realizing that the existing chaotic health nonsystem must be placed in more integrated enterpreneural hands to be a good market for heavy computer hardware, or for sophisticated private consultation services. Thus, for a variety of reasons, national corporate leaders are encouraging Einstein-Montefiore's rationalization of the Bronx.

A natural law of many well-promoted medical demonstration projects is that the further one gets from the project's patients, the better the project looks. Einstein-

Montefiore is perhaps as much or more involved in service than any other major medical center in the nation—but its experiments in rationalizing the health care system are not exceptions to this law. For all its declarations about social commitment, the empire has barely scratched the surface of meeting the desperate needs in its region, especially in the south Bronx.

The south Bronx is a disaster area for personal and environmental health. Its proportion of health services users of dependent age (over sixty-five or under sixteen) is the largest in the city. Its general dependence on municipal hsopitals, general service baby deliveries, and public ambulance service is the greatest in the city. Its rates of too-late or nonexistent prenatal care are among the worst for municipal hospitals. The area's venereal disease, chronic disease, and infant and maternal mortality rates are among the highest in the city; early findings of recent studies reveal the city's highest rates of lead poisoning in children; dilapidated housing, garbage-heaped streets, and polluted air are as serious as anywhere in the city. Certain areas of the south Bronx have less community-physician coverage than the physician-to-black-citizen ratio in Mississippi. One-third of the borough's residents must go to Manhattan for hospitalization, even in emergencies, primarily because of the shortage of medical resources in the south Bronx. Clearly, without massive amounts of direct public disaster area relief, the people of this area face a catastrophic social breakdown.

When confronted with the medical and environmental wreckage of the south Bronx, the empire's promoters point with pride to their two magnaminous ghetto demonstration projects—the Lincoln Mental Health Center and the O.E.O.-funded Martin Luther King Health Center.

But what these projects actually demonstrate is that isolated gestures, however showy, are bound to fail. Together, the two projects probably serve no more than 30,000 people out of at least 700,000 in the south Bronx area. The health center's expansion has been checked by its uniquely high costs (estimates are in the neighborhood of one hundred dollars per patient-visit!), which partially reflect the program's luxurious anthropological and sociological research component, the business of which is to convert services rendered into academically impressive data and reports. "If this health center demonstrates anything," said one local public official, "it is that such a program cannot possibly be duplicated." The mental health center is a far more striking demonstration of the empire's inability to deliver public service in return for public funds. A 1969 investigation by the National Institute of Mental Health revealed that hundreds of thousands of federal dollars earmarked for mental health services had been simply absorbed by the center of the empire for other uses (see chapter VI).

To most of the residents of the Bronx, however, these demonstrations are not visible enough to be a source of scandal. The poor and working people of the Bronx rely on the empire-affiliated municipal hospitals for their health services, and it is only through these hospitals that they know the empire. Einstein-Montefiore's claims for its boroughwide network of affiliations are staggering. They cite, with some justification, improvements in the number of physician staff and in the educational level at the municipal-affiliate hospitals, and increased specialty services. Whether the affiliation-spawned proliferation of subspecialty clinics at the empire-controlled public hospitals is a gain for the patients, however, is not so clear. The fragmentation of the clinics along narrow academic lines (hematology, genetics, etc.) means increasingly fragmented care for the patient—more wasted clinic visits, more unnecessary diagnostic procedures (sometimes performed for research purposes), more lost medical records, and an ever more desperate search for the right doctor at the right time for a specific problem. Thus what the empire-promoter calls a "broad spectrum of new services" turns out to be an unscannable spectrum for the patient.

The affiliation programs have achieved some new administrative contact among the various hospitals. But there has been far too little real service coordination. There is no continuity of medical records between the empire's hospitals, and sometimes not even much cooperation. For instance, if a patient is referred from Lincoln to Jacobi for specialized treatment, Lincoln does not send his medical record with him, nor does Jacobi bother to send Lincoln a record of what happened during specialty treatment. Women who have received prenatal care at Lincoln are often sent out of the empire, to Manhattan's New York Hospital, to deliver—again with only minimal medical records. None of this is helped, of course, by the fact that many of the patients are Spanish-speaking, and are shunted from clinic to clinic, hospital to hospital, with little or no comprehensible explanation.

Few of the people who rely on the empire for health services know of its liberal, rational image in Washington, or its exaggerated claims to service with the downtown public health bureaucracy. They know that Montefiore and Einstein's College Hospital are the "good" hospitals— for someone else's use. They know that Lincoln and Morrisania are second-rate, dumping grounds for the poor and uninteresting patients rejected by Montefiore and Einstein. And in the south Bronx people still call Lincoln "the slaughterhouse." When striking Lincoln hospital workers were threatened with dispersal by the police in the spring of 1969, one worker commented wryly, "They (the administration) don't know their own power—they just have to threaten us with violence. If we thought we were going to be injured this close to Lincoln, and be taken there, we'd all throw up our hands."

As this and other medical empires are under more and more public attack for their failure to deliver, even with what they've got, the promoters become all the more radical at laying the blame elsewhere. They cite the city's bureaucratic red tape; severe national underfinancing (and misregulation) of research, care, and education; and, of course, the general social chaos of the nation. These exogenous difficulties are, of course, part of the story. But the empire-promoters are seldom able to face their own responsibility honestly, and to say, as Pogo was once quoted, "We have seen the enemy and it is us."

VI

EMPIRES AT WORK:
THE CASE OF THE COMMUNITY
MENTAL HEALTH CENTERS

The mental health marketplace looks, at first glance, strikingly similar to the medical care marketplace. Much of the manpower is still scattered in private offices, though increasingly it is becoming concentrated in the psychiatry departments of medical schools and in major voluntary hospitals. For most people, basic ambulatory and preventive services are financially, if not geographically, inaccessible, although free hospitalization awaits at the terminal stages of illness. The analogy to the medical marketplace is particularly clear in New York City. The city mental health agency, the Community Mental Health Board (C.M.H.B.), in a caricature of the City Hospital Department's affiliation program, confines its activities to writing contracts with private providers, and provides no services itself. The few mental health services that are operated directly by the city, like those in the city hospitals, serve chiefly the poor and the acute emergencies. In fact, both city hospitals and city-run mental hospitals hark back to a common ancestor—the town lunatic asylum.

This, then, is the mental health care scene today in New

York City and many other urban centers: For the poor, there are no mental health services—only various degrees of detention and isolation. For the middle-class patient, facilities exist, but it is questionable whether any of them will be interested in the particular set of problems the patient presents at the time he presents them. From a public policy point of view, the system is irrational, expensive, and grossly wasteful of manpower.

As in the physical health field, there is growing government concern about the disorganization of mental health services in the face of mounting demand. And, as in physical health, public efforts to spread mental health services around rely almost wholly on the imagination and good will of the private strongholds of professional manpower. At the federal level, wellspring of much corporate medicine, vast sums were earmarked in the mid-1960s for local experiments in mental health—community mental health centers.

President Kennedy's Community Mental Health Center Act of 1963 was heralded as a bold new approach to mental illness. Actually, it represented little more than the application of some common-sense principles of public health to the traditionally murky area of mental health. The idea was that mental illness, like other illnesses, could be checked by intervention at early stages. By making comprehensive mental health services available in residential communities, millions of people could potentially be headed off from lengthy incarcerations in state institutions. The federal government would provide a share of construction and staffing money, asking only that the centers provide a full range of services (inpatient, outpatient, emergency, etc.) and relate to a community somewhere between 75,000 and 200,000 in population. Community participation in the planning and operation of the centers was also mandated, not so much as an invitation to community control, but as a public relations measure. Questions about what kinds of illnesses the centers would deal with, how they would be staffed, what degree of community participation they would feature, etc., were all left to local public health agencies to resolve.

C.M.H.B. was the New York City agency which found itself charged with the task of translating the community mental health center concept into a brick-and-mortar program. C.M.H.B. is the most reticent, least publicized of New York City's health agencies. It presents no public profile of buildings or programs, operates with a small and relatively placid staff, and has usually remained aloof from the routine crises common to other city agencies, including other health agencies. Unlike the appointed commissioners of other city agencies, who report directly to the Mayor, the Commissioner of Mental Health reports to an unpaid nine-member board, which in turn is responsible to the Mayor and to the State Department of Mental Hygiene. The reason for this unusual arrangement was that C.M.H.B. was created through state legislation rather than directly by the city government. The 1954 State Mental Hygiene Law had made available state matching funds for local public and private mental health services, and authorized the establishment of local city and county C.M.H.B.s to administer the funds.

There was no reason why C.M.H.B. could not have used state monies to operate its own programs, but an early Board decision established the policy of contracting out for all direct services. Thus C.M.H.B. is essentially no more than a conduit, passing on government funds to a wide range of uncoordinated private mental health facilities.

From top to bottom, C.M.H.B. is characterized by a severe case of conflict-of-interest. Except for two *ex officio* public officials, C.M.H.B.'s elite Board is fairly evenly divided between representatives of the city's two major philanthropic organizations, Catholic Charities and the Federation of Jewish Philanthropies, which together dominate the city's sectarian health and hospital facilities. All of the mental health facilities under the egis of these two philanthropic organizations receive public funds through C.M.H.B. and collectively absorb a large percentage of C.M.H.B.'s total outlay for private agencies. Other affiliations of C.M.H.B. members include the institutional centers of some of the city's most patrician empires—the Columbia University Medical Center and the Cornell University Medical Center. Ties to the private, C.M.H.B.-funded mental health sector are just as tight at the staff level in C.M.H.B. Several middle-echelon C.M.H.B. staffers interviewed in late 1968 were found to work part-time for private agencies receiving C.M.H.B. funds. Not surprisingly, considering these sources of recruitment, C.M.H.B.'s staff presents a white, middle-aged, well-fed face. In mid-1968, C.M.H.B. had only three nonwhite employees (out of 170) above the clerical level.

C.M.H.B.'s overall policies have been generally consistent with the interests of the staff and Board, and with the interests of the institutions which they represent. A disproportionate share of funds goes to voluntary agencies—which usually charge fees, and employ other, even more direct mechanisms of selecting middle-class, articulate patients—as compared to city-run services which serve only the indigent. For instance, in 1961, city-run clinics were handling seventy-eight percent of the city's total psychiatric outpatient admissions and receiving forty-five percent of the C.M.H.B. funds for clinic care. Voluntary agencies under contract to C.M.H.B. were handling twenty-two percent of the admissions and receiving fifty-four percent of the funds. The disproportion has, if anything, increased since that time. Voluntary agencies receiving C.M.H.B. funds have been virtually unregulated, with contracts specifying little more than the name of the agency and its budget. About five new voluntary agencies have gained C.M.H.B. contracts each year, amounting to a total of sixty-six such fortunate agencies in 1968, but it has proved nearly impossible for a black- or Puerto Rican-run agency to gain C.M.H.B. support.

From the start, C.M.H.B.'s interpretation of the Community Mental Health Centers Act clearly reflected the needs and interests of the city's medical empires. First, C.M.H.B. required that all community mental health centers had to be "affiliated with a teaching hospital or medical school, closely related and located within a reasonable distance to a general hospital," i.e., community mental health centers had to fall administratively and geographically within one of the city's medical empires. Secondly, C.M.H.B. tended to see mental health centers almost exclusively as new buildings, although the cheaper and more flexible interpretation of them as networks of services was well within the law, and would have required about ten years less to implement. But nothing, of course, could have been more attractive to an expansionist medical empire than a new, ten- or twenty-million-dollar, publicly-financed building.

In 1965, C.M.H.B. staff came up with a "master plan" for covering the entire city with community mental health centers. The city was divided into fifty-one areas tailored to fit federal population requirements (between 75,000 and

200,000 residents). Each of the fifty-one catchment areas, as they were called, was designed to cover the widest possible range of socioeconomic conditions—a feature which not only pleased the integrationists in C.M.H.B., but also assured that no community mental health center would be too heavily burdened with "inarticulate," "deprived" patients. Once the maps were drawn, C.M.H.B. saw no further need for planning: all catchment areas were to have community mental health centers, but in no particular order of priority. The only task was to find the institutions to staff them.

In its early efforts to sell community mental health centers, C.M.H.B. never strayed far from the centers of the city's seven medical empires (see chapter XVI). With maps in hand, C.M.H.B. staff dashed out to promote the program to medical schools and teaching hospitals—as a first step, Columbia was asked to take Washington Heights, Einstein to take the Bronx, and New York University was asked to take the Bellevue area on the lower east side. C.M.H.B.'s promotion of centers was reminiscent of the Department of Hospitals' earlier efforts to enlist private institutions for the hospital affiliation program: the private institutions were sometimes reticent but yielded to the promise of staff salaries, a new building, and the unbeatable argument, "only *you* have the expertise to do it."

The Columbia and Einstein empires each bought the community mental health center idea for their own, very different reasons. Columbia wanted space to expand its existing Freudian analytical-training and drug-oriented research programs. Einstein leaped at the chance for federal funds to enable bright young staff men to do their thing in "the community." If their thing meant new, socially oriented "demonstration" projects, so much the better, since these in turn could be the basis for further grant-hustling and talent recruitment. Programmatic considerations aside, Einstein was interested in any new public funds, no matter how earmarked, which could be siphoned off to shore up existing mental health programs in the empire— at Einstein, Montefiore, Bronx Municipal, and Bronx State hospitals.

*   *   *

Einstein College of Medicine-Yeshiva University didn't even wait for new buildings to be constructed before setting up its two centers in the Bronx: Soundview-Throgs Neck-Tremont Community Mental Health Center and the Lincoln Hospital Community Mental Health Services. Both centers are linked for staffing and backup services to other institutions within the empire—primarily to the psychiatric wards at Bronx Municipal Hospital and Bronx State (mental) Hospital. The empire has encouraged, in its own words, a global approach to psychiatry which includes centrally-controlled shifts of staff and funds from institution to institution.

The Einstein venture in Soundview–Throgs Neck–Tremont was never a bold, new approach, but a continuation of a pre-1963 program, dressed up to meet the requirements for federal community mental health centers money. The center is not a building, but a concept—an administrative network linking Einstein-run mental health services in the catchment area with the wards in Einstein-affiliated hospitals. If there is any difference between the Soundview-Throgs Neck program before and after it became a community mental health center, it is probably that as a center, it is more smoothly managed. Patients and patients' medical records are not as likely to be lost in transit between the three mental health clinics in the Soundview-Throgs Neck area and the distant wards at Bronx State.

Are the people of Soundview–Throgs Neck–Tremont grateful for this new convenience? It is unlikely that very many of the residents are even aware of the two million dollar program in their midst. The center has minimized preventive services, out-reach, and special action programs, preferring to concentrate on the few "really sick" persons who surface from the population. The center's director, an Einstein man, regards "community control-niks," socially oriented professionals, and the like as poachers. If the community wants to get involved in mental health, it should get a grant to do its own thing—far from his medical show.

Einstein reserved its showcase community mental health center for Lincoln Hospital, a municipal hospital which, along with the blighted south Bronx area which surrounds it, has been rapidly decaying for two decades. The south Bronx, a transposed and expanded version of the waterfront slums of San Juan, is distinguished by the highest crime and addiction rates in New York. Mental health services may not be what the south Bronx needed most, but it got them, starting in 1963, to the tune of $1.5 million, expanding to $4.5 million in 1968. On paper, the Lincoln community mental health center was the most lavish, most socially oriented mental health program in the city, if not the nation. Einstein boasted of the center's innovative projects in addiction, rehabilitation services, community action, and out-reach. Not until the center's workers revolted in 1969 was it revealed by a federal investigation that much of this program was non-existent—the money had been drained off to sponsor other imperial enterprises.

In June, 1969, investigations by Lincoln mental health workers and federal investigators from the National Institute of Mental Health demonstrated that Einstein's global approach was a one-way street leading directly to the empire's coffers.

The empire had skimmed off over $500,000 in overhead alone since 1965. Hidden benefits in the form of (unrelated) staff salaries, new positions, and additional factilities were accumulated through padding. Not only did Einstein not pour personnel time into the Lincoln program, but they took an additional $45,000 per year to pay for a battery of accountants, bookkeepers, etc. to work at Einstein.

It was not unusual for Lincoln Mental Health Center to wait for up to six months for its money to be passed on by Einstein. An administrator working closely with Einstein says the reason for the delay was not the work load or lack of administrative capacity, but that Einstein had greatly underestimated the deficit to be incurred from its own College Hospital; and Einstein simply preferred to use the Lincoln money, rather than dig into its own capital funds.

Bronx State Hospital, another affiliate of Einstein, also took its share. During fiscal year 1968–69, $25,000 went to supplement the drug addiction ward at Bronx State where Lincoln Mental Health Center was to be allotted twenty-four beds for detoxification. The doctor in charge of the service allowed only four beds to be utilized. More outrageous, was the disappearance of an additional $137,000 which was to be used to hire a "liaison staff" for Bronx State's eighty-bed Lincoln ward. Only one psychiatrist was hired, and even he did not relate directly to Lincoln Mental Health Center.

Three neighborhood mental health units at $70,000 each were to have been established, and only one was in existence by mid-1969. Similarly, a mandated $64,000 staff for outpatient care was nonexistent. Even more spectacular was the case of the phantom $372,000 partial hospitalization program which was supposed to provide weekend, evening, and daytime services.

Though $136,000 was provided for establishing a psychiatric emergency room service, sporadic emergency care was provided through the general Lincoln hospital emergency room. One need only realize that the Lincoln emergency room is the second busiest in the nation to appreciate the insanity of the situation. When a government investigating team visited the emergency room, it found that the psychiatric staff was not even present—only available on call. The mental health emergency service had neither a telephone listing nor a telephone answering service.

The official document prepared by the federal investigating team, an open letter from the National Institute of Mental Health to New York City's Commissioner of Mental Health, dated July 9, 1969, found that "an identifiable community mental health center . . . does not exist fiscally, administratively or programmatically." But after scolding Yeshiva University (and its fiscal intermediary, Albert Einstein) for the most blatant breaches of contract, the officials made no move to fund a more responsible, alternative structure. In the meantime, the Einstein Department of Psychiatry—which would like to preserve its year-old residency program at Lincoln—made its position more secure by creating a Lincoln Hospital Department of Psychiatry. With this arrangement, if the community mental health center fails, only the community can lose. Traditional, teaching-oriented inpatient services will go on at the Lincoln Department of Psychiatry. As have been the empire's paternalistic attitude toward its Lincoln colony in the past —he who giveth, can taketh away.

*   *   *

The Columbia University College of Physicians and Surgeons empire will probably never be charged with malfeasance as was the Einstein empire, because its elaborate plan for a community mental health center never got off the drawing boards. The public can only speculate that, had the black and Puerto Rican community not stood in its way, Columbia would be well on its way to developing a human laboratory for its own research and training priorities—with mental health services to the surrounding Washington Heights-West Harlem community running a very poor third.

In 1967, when Columbia first began to discuss the prospect of a community mental health center with C.M.H.B., probably few residents of the catchment area were even aware that the Columbia Medical Center offered mental health services. In the academic psychiatric world, however, Columbia is internationally famous as the best Columbia's psychiatric resources consist of a loose complex of four separate and discrete elements, linked administratively and through personnel overlap. At the core is the Department of Psychiatry, which trains medical students and offers psychiatric residencies, and is headed by a recent past president of the American Psychiatric Association. For higher training, there is the Psychoanalytic Clinic for Research and Training, which is not a clinic at all, but one of the three top psychoanalytic insti-

tutes in New York City, well-known for its hard-line
Freudian orientation. Access to patients for these two
training and research centers is provided by Presbyterian
Hospital's clinic and the Psychiatric Institute, an affiliated
182-bed state research and training hospital.

As in the medical center generally, psychiatric research
and training come first, while service admittedly takes
lower priority. Even C.M.H.B. acknowledged that Columbia "has been able to provide only limited service facilities to the people of Washington Heights." Since much of
the training is aimed at the production of psychiatrists and
analysts for private practice, what service is offered tends
to be selective for the kind of middle-class, articulate patients who are believed to be susceptible to conventional
individual therapy. Thus at the Psychiatric Institute, only
one sixty-bed floor is reserved for community people,
while the rest serve mainly middle-class patients from
throughout the city. Therapy on the community floor is
heavily drug-dependent, in line with the Psychiatric Institute's active involvement in testing for drug companies.
As for the low-income Washington Heights community,
a high-ranking faculty member in the Columbia Department of Psychiatry wrote in 1964: "A local community
adjacent to the medical center has been delineated as a lab
for long term studies of various therapeutic techniques. .
. . The population of the Washington Heights Health District, with a population of 269,000 (sic), constitutes the
'laboratory community.'"

Long before the community mental health center issue
surfaced, Columbia's relationship to the Washington
Heights-West Harlem community had been growing
tenser, while its relationship to C.M.H.B. had been grow-

ing more intimate. Community resentment focussed on Columbia's expansionist real estate policies in the over-crowded slum areas, and was in no way softened by the empire's medical policies, which favored research, education, and private patient care over community service. But to the downtown offices of C.M.H.B., Columbia was a close friend and colleague. A Columbia faculty member has, since 1964, held a seat on C.M.H.B.'s elite, non-salaried board, while a Columbia associate professor held (until 1967) the top staff position (commissioner) at C.M.H.B. The Columbia-C.M.H.B. relationship was further cemented in the mid-sixties by joint research and education projects, such as survey of the public image of mental health, and a C.M.H.B. residency program for Columbia trainees in administrative psychiatry.

When the community mental center program got underway in 1966, Columbia was not only assured a center, but one to be built entirely with public funds. (Two other voluntary hospitals in New York put up much of their own construction money for centers.) After working out an informal agreement with Columbia's Division of Community Psychiatry, C.M.H.B.'s commissioner proceeded to enter the project—the city's first—into C.M.H.B.'s 1966–67 budget for new construction. Lest the C.M.H.B. board balk at the eighteen-million-dollar request, city Hospital Commissioner Trussell made an unprecedented personal appearance before the board to plead for the community mental health center. His efforts were instrumental in pushing the Columbia center over the wire. (Three weeks after his appeal to C.M.H.B.'s board, the Commissioner resigned his city post and headed back to the deanship of the Columbia School of Public Health, which, along with the Columbia Department of Psychiatry, jointly administers the Division of Community Psychiatry.)

Within months, the architects (a private firm under contract to the city) and Columbia planners unveiled their plan for what was heralded by C.M.H.B. as a model community mental health center. The plan was never made public and was, in fact, later suppressed by both Columbia and C.M.H.B. But because of its sumptuous proportions, it has become legendary in city planning and budgeting circles. It included 407 offices for the private use of Columbia psychiatrists! The actual services, if not an afterthought, were at best far from innovative. At the core was a good-sized hospital—two hundred patient beds. The other federally mandated services appeared to have been designed from a federal how-to-do-it guidebook with little attention to whatever special needs or tastes the community might have. There were a token ten beds for drug addicts, a slightly smaller service for alcoholics, and no program whatever to utilize the supportive services of existing local social service agencies.

Struck by the probable expense of this monumental community mental health center, the state's Department of Mental Hygiene did not challenge the 407 private offices, but only suggested that two hundred beds (which in theory justified the office space) were more than enough for two catchment areas. The state proposed that the Inwood catchment area be attached to Washington Heights-West Harlem for a total catchment area population of 281,330, more than enough to stock the two hundred beds. In order to conform to the federal law limiting catchment populations to 200,000, the Columbia community mental health center's plans were revised to provide for two separate but equal sets of services under the one roof: one set for the predominantly black and Puerto Rican southern Washington Heights and West Harlem, and another for the mostly white northern Washington Heights and Inwood.

Columbia jumped at the chance to redefine its catchment area. From the beginning of the discussion of the mental health center, Columbia had expressed a preference for reaching northward to the white areas, rather than serving the black and Puerto Rican Washington Heights-West Harlem. If C.M.H.B. were going to insist that the mental health center serve the blacks and Puerto Ricans of southern Washington Heights and West Harlem, the lower-class clientele would at least be counterbalanced by white Inwoodites. And, most important of all, the move preserved the 407 offices which could easily house a couch for every therapist in Columbia's Department of Psychiatry, as well as provide room for research.

Black and Puerto Rican leaders of the Washington Heights-West Harlem community greeted the idea of a Columbia-run community mental health center with immediate hostility. Community activists countered Columbia's plans with a vision of a mental health center as a street-level beachhead against addiction and alcoholism, and as springboard for an attack on all the environmental and institutional causes of distress. When the Columbia two-entrance plan leaked out, resentment mounted and became more widespread. The final blow was the announcement of the location Columbia and C.M.H.B. had selected for the center—the site of the Audubon Ballroom, scene of Malcolm X's assassination and, to blacks, a national shrine. At a 1968 community meeting called by Columbia to satisfy federal requirements for community involvement in mental health center planning, black and Puerto Rican residents seized the podium, denounced Columbia's plans, and declared that henceforth the community would plan for its own mental health services.

This incident came close to becoming a severe political embarrassment to C.M.H.B., and hence to the mayor. In the weeks that followed the community "takeover", as it was called, C.M.H.B. went through some painful introspection. First, it hired a black social worker to fill the new post of community liaison. Then, impressed by the evident urgency of community demand for mental health services, C.M.H.B. reversed its former policy and decided to encourage the development of new community mental health centers which were not new buildings, but "integrated networks of services." However, C.M.H.B. did not alter its on-going plans for construction of fifteen new centers. Without them, it is doubtful whether C.M.H.B. would have had any notion of how to lure most of the city's medical empires into community mental health center programs.

Columbia, for one, was not going to step down into the streets with any loose network of services. Its response to the community revolt and to the less cooperative stance of C.M.H.B. was to gradually disentangle itself from any commitment to mental health services in the Washington Heights-West Harlem area. In an October 1968 speech at a meeting of the American Psychiatric Association, Columbia's director of psychiatry questioned whether psychiatrists should support continued federal funding to the community mental health centers program. He further questioned whether it was realistic to ever hope for the kind of redistribution of services implied by the Community Mental Health Centers Act, given the priorities of the empires. "There are clinical and organizational patterns, not always recognized, that militate against what we might consider the rational distribution of medical care of any kind, and perhaps especially of mental health care," he was quoted as saying.

Later, in his 1969 Presidential Address to the American Psychiatric Association, Kolb stated that if the mental health establishment had a social responsibility at all, it was to prevent, rather than to foment, community action. "Administrators and deliverers of mental health services will have to sharpen their perception and recognition of their responsibilities in maintaining social homeostasis. They bear a social responsibility much in the same way as the courts *and other law enforcement agencies* do in the support of a healthy community environment for all." (Emphasis added.)

By mid-1969, Columbia had withdrawn all its plans for a community mental health center and made it known to C.M.H.B. that it would take much more than a 407-room office building to reawaken its interest.

The bloom is off the community mental health centers program in New York City. After the confrontation in Washington Heights, Columbia simply picked up its academic robes and retreated to its fortress-like domain on the edge of the Hudson River. And, after its embarrassment at Lincoln, Einstein has begun to retrench to the safety of its more established hospital outposts. Other private institutions in the city are reevaluating their plans for community mental health centers or, like New York University Medical Center, are gerrymandering their catchment areas to exclude potentially demanding black and Puerto Rican neighborhoods. C.M.H.B., recently brought under more careful government scrutiny, and renamed Depart-

ment of Mental Health, has become more cautious about
its projections of high quality, convenient mental health
services for all.

Yet at the outset of the community mental health center
planning, New York had everything in its favor—a largesse of psychiatric resources, a powerful public mental
health agency, and a galaxy of willing medical empires.
The program in New York was entrusted by the government to some of the most prestigious medical empires in
the nation, and to the extent that the program has failed,
they have failed. Columbia and Einstein molded the flexible community mental health centers concept to fit their
institutional needs—for space, for funds, for grant-worthy
"demonstrations." If these needs did not correspond to the
needs of the service-starved "target populations," so much
the worse for the target populations. The empires had
other things on their agendas.

VII

THE MEDICAL-INDUSTRIAL COMPLEX

Ever since Florence Nightingale, medical care has had an aura of selflessness and self-imposed poverty. The great modern hospital center, for instance, projects itself as a nonprofit institution where "the few toil ceaselessly that the many might live." But behind the facade of the helpless sick and the dedicated healers lies the 1960s' greatest gold rush, a booming "health industry" churning out more than $2.5 billion a year by 1969 in after-tax profits.

In 1969 the nation spent over $62 billion on medical care, a figure up more than eleven percent from the previous year and twice the 1960 total. Six billion dollars of this flowed into the hands of the drug companies, almost ten billion went to the companies that sell doctors and hospitals everything from bed linen to electrocardiographs. $3.5 billion was spent on "proprietary" (profit-making) hospitals and nursing homes. The nation purchases six billion dollars worth of commercial health insurance, and construction companies built about two billion dollars worth of hospitals. Additional billions were raked in by private physicians. The health industry is big business, profitable business, and booming business. Stockbroker Goodbody and Company clued in its customers in its May 1969 Monthly Letter: "Steady growth of the health industry . . . is as certain as anything can be."

The great boom of the 1960s in the health industries was largely the product of government subsidization of the market. For years the government has directly or indirectly fed dollars into the gaping pockets of the dealers in human disease. In addition to direct payments for health care, for educating health manpower, and for hospital construction, it has granted tax deductions to individuals for their medical expenses, making their health dollars cheaper. It has expanded the purchasing power of the so-called nonprofit hospitals by granting them tax exemptions, and, until recently, by exempting them from minimum wage or labor relations laws. It has directly supported basic biological and chemical research to the tune of billions of dollars, and has sponsored dramatic advances in electronics. These basic technologies underlie many of the most profitable sectors of the health industry. And in 1966, the biggest government subsidy of all—Medicare and Medicaid—got going. By 1969, federal, state, and local governments directly picked up more than a third of the tab for the nation's health needs, and all signals were go for a steadily increasing government-guaranteed market. One likely mechanism: government subsidized national health insurance, to underwrite the entire medical care market (see chapter XII).

Only a small part of the new money being spent on health, however, has gone to improve health care. For instance, community hospitals spent sixteen percent more money in 1968 than they did in 1967. But they provided only 3.3 percent more days of inpatient care and 3.7 percent more outpatient visits. (Nobody noticed any thirteen percent increase in the quality of care). A large fraction of the new money for the health care delivery system has, for all social purposes, simply vanished—as inflated costs for drugs, supplies and equipment, and as profits for doctors and hospitals.

From the outset, the aim of the health industry—the private companies which supply, equip, finance, build for, and (sometimes) manage the health delivery system—is not to promote the general well-being, but to exploit existing profitable markets and create new ones. Its emphasis, then, is not on products and services which would improve basic health care for the great mass of consumers, but on what are essentially luxury items: electronic thermometers, hyperbaric chambers, hospitals which specialize in elective surgery for the rich, expensive combination drugs. Under the pressure of the industry's barrage of packaged technology, the health care delivery system is increasingly distorted towards high-cost, low-utilization, inpatient services.

Much of the money which flows through the delivery system to the health industry's drug and hospital supply and equipment companies never returns to the delivery system in any medically useful form, or in any form at all. A good five to ten percent is raked off directly as profits, and these by and large vanish into the larger economy, going to stockholders and going to finance the companies' expansions into other enterprises. More and more of the health industry firms are conglomerates, whose holdings in drugs or hospital supplies help finance their acquisitions in cosmetics, catering, or pet food.

Profits are only part of the story however. There is no way of auditing the health industry companies to determine how much of their "costs" are actually socially necessary. Prices are high, the health companies claim, not on account of profits, but because of the enormous cost of research, skilled manpower, meeting exacting standards, etc. But how much of the industry's research goes into a needless and dangerously confusing proliferation of marginally different products—like drugs which differ only in flavor, electronic equipment which differs only in console design? How much goes to plan the planned obsolescence in expensive hospital hardware? How much of the costs go for the design of appealing packaging? How much for multi-million-dollar advertising and promotion campaigns? Money spent on these causes is not simply wasted. The needless proliferation of dazzlingly advertised and packaged products is a health hazard. It prevents the buyer, whether he is a doctor, a hospital administrator, or a patient, from making informed choices among products and mystifies him to the point where he will accept unquestioningly the industry's definition of what he needs and what he must pay for it.

Drugs

The drug industry likes to think of itself as a sort of public service, dispensing life and comfort and at the same time upholding the American, free enterprise way. *Forbes* magazine, which likes to think of itself as the "capitalist tool," much more honestly describes the drug industry as "one of the biggest crap games in U.S. industry." Any way you cut it, the drug industry is big and on the way to being bigger:

> ——six billion dollars worth of drugs (prescription and non-prescription) were sold in 1969, $6.5 billion will be sold in 1970, and so on, increasing at about nine percent a year,
> ——there are 700 drug firms. Control is concentrated in the top fifteen, who sell more than half of all drugs,
> ——200,000 people are employed by drug companies all

over the world. 100,000 of these are Americans and 20,000 of them are the "detail men" who push prescription pills to private doctors,

——the American drug industry is worldwide. Foreign sales are growing faster than domestic, as drug companies expand their foreign subsidiaries. The two leading drug imperialists are Pfizer, with forty-eight percent of its business abroad, and Merck, with thirty-seven percent. Industry-wide more than one-quarter of sales are abroad,

——the industry spends one-and-a-half billion dollars a year on sales and content, twenty-five cents out of every sales dollar, and more than three times as much as it spends on its much-heralded research and development effort.

What makes the drug industry the "biggest crap game," however, is its profits. For the last ten years, the drug industry has held either first, second, or third place among all U.S. industries in terms of profitability, out-distancing such obvious moneymakers as the cosmetics, aerospace, recreation, and entertainment industries.

But the drug industry has seen better days. Earlier leaps in profits grew out of major breakthroughs: antibiotics in the late '40s, tranquilizers in the late '50s and early '60s, and birth control pills in the early and mid-'60s. Nothing big has come along since "the pill," and even it is something of a disappointment. Even before the 1970 Senate hearings on pill safety, efforts to push the pill beyond the twenty percent of eligible women who now use it had been checked by growing mutters about annoying and sometimes lethal side effects. "We're in a trough right now," says a top Merck man, and some companies are beginning to wonder whether it's worth gambling on another wave of wonder drugs.

According to the industry's own probably inflated estimates, a really new drug takes about ten years and seven million dollars worth of research. Hence more and more new drugs are not new at all. Over half of those released in the last ten years are what are called "me too" drugs: minor chemical modifications of old drugs, combinations of old drugs, old drugs released in chewable form, time capsule form, half-dose form, in handy dispensers, and so on in endless, meaningless elaboration. Meanwhile, some of the old best-sellers are threatened with patent expirations and antitrust suits. Parke-Davis had become too dependent on chloromycetin. Bad publicity about the drug's side effects followed by the expiration of the antibiotic's patent a couple of years ago caused a decline in the company's profitability. Similarly, Pfizer has lost an antitrust suit which will loosen its grip on tetracycline. Overall drug industry profits slipped below ten percent of sales in 1968 for the first time in years. (That's still way ahead of most industries.)

Then, as if the drug companies didn't have enough problems of their own, the federal government has shown increasing signs of being serious about regulating drug costs and quality. The Kefauver investigations into drug prices and the resulting federal drug law amendments had drug companies, by their own admission, running scared in the early sixties. The stiffer scrutiny of new drugs required by the 1962 law caused a sharp drop in the rate at which new products were introduced, and pushed many companies to expand abroad in countries where drug testing and marketing laws are more permissive.

But the most potentially far-reaching affront to the drug companies' independence was Medicare. Drug companies knew from the start that a healthy chunk of Medicare funds would find its way to their pockets. What they feared was that there might be some strings attached. The Pharmaceutical Manufacturers Association, in its right wing public relations throwaway "Medicine at Work," editorialized in early 1965:

> What is the logic in socializing medical care [via Medicare] when health insurance programs can function so effectively and are expanding every day, in fact already covering most of our citizens? . . . If private initiative disappears there may never be enough time to repair the damage that will ensue.

But a few months later the Pharmaceutical Manufacturers Association, at their national convention, spent a whole day in seminars on Medicare. When they emerged, the *New York Times* reported with cautious optimism that "some companies have accepted the fact that Medicare is here and with it has come a new opportunity for the industry."

Even though they reluctantly accepted Medicare (and, of course, Medicare money for their pills), the drug companies saw trouble ahead. Like the A.M.A., the drug industry knows that government subsidy can lead to government scrutiny. Drug costs are a big bill to swallow, and have already become the subject of repeated Congressional inquiry. If the government role in financing medical care expands beyond Medicare and the ruins of Medicaid, the government might begin to insist on generic drugs (as opposed to much more expensive but chemically identical brand-name drugs), price-setting, or other forms of profit-cutting regulation.

When the neighborhood pusher feels the heat coming down on him, he begins to turn to new, but related, rackets. So with the drug companies, menaced by real or imagined regulation, the answer has been to diversify into anything for which their technology and marketing skills prepare them. As if by free association, drug companies have been turning to cosmetics, chemicals, hospital supplies, and electronic equipment for hospitals. American Cyanamid (which owns Lederle Labs) now owns Breck Shampoo. Pfizer has bought Coty, Barbasol, Pacquin, and Desitin (baby powders and oils). Richardson-Merrill acquired Clearasil; Smith, Kline and French has Sea and Ski. Syntex, Upjohn, and Merck are all reaching into chemicals. Upjohn, Searle and Smith, Kline and French are all involved in medical electronics, with Searle, for instance, betting on Medidata, which makes computers for futuristic mechanized mass screening devices. Parke-Davis and Abbott and Cutter Labs are getting into the booming hospital supplies industry.

All this diversification by the once staid drug manufacturers does not represent a flight from drugs. Prescription drugs remain the most profitable line of the diversified companies, and the drug habit, once established, is hard to break. In fact, the most interesting trend in the drug industry is not diversification of the old guard, but the influx of new industries, all potential drug addicts. Chemical companies are leading the way. Dow Chemicals, of Saran Wrap and napalm fame, began buying up small drug companies in 1960, and is now a major contender in the measles vaccine market. Other chemical newcomers are 3M (formerly Minnesota Mining and Manufacturing, the conglomerate which makes, among other things, Scotch Tape), Rohm and Haas, Union Carbide, Malinckrodt and DuPont. Cosmetic and soap companies, such as Bristol-Meyers, Colgate-Palmolive, and Helene Curtis are not far behind in the rush for the drug markets. Revlon now owns U.S. Vitamin and Pharmaceuticals; Cheeseborough, Pond has acquired Pertussin. One other industry which is being invaded by the drug firms has begun a counteroffensive—the medical supplies industry. Baxter, Becton-Dickinson, and Johnson and Johnson have all bought into the drug industry.

You don't have to be a member of the chemical-drug-cosmetics axis to get in on the drug action. For intance, American Home Products, Inc., maker of Boyardee Foods, Gulden's Mustard and Gay-pet products for animals also serves up nonprescription drugs such as Preparation H, Quiet World (a tranquilizer), and Sudden Action (breath freshener), and has become a big shot in the ethical drug world, owning Wyeth Labs as well as several smaller drug companies. Then there's Squibb-Beechnut which makes gum, baby foods, candy, coffee, pastry, airline meals, and operates drive-ins and snack bars, in addition to making prescription drugs. Anybody who makes anything which can be swallowed, inhaled, absorbed, or applied would like to make drugs—and vice versa.

Hospital Supplies and Equipment

The story of the growth of the hospital supplies industry is the story of the explosive growth of the hospital as the central institution in the delivery of health care in America. In 1950 the nation spent $3.8 billion on hospital care. By 1965, the figure had risen to $13.8 billion, and in 1969, three years after Medicare and Medicaid, hospital expenditures were running at a $20 billion a year clip. About $7.5 billion of this went for goods and services. Much of it is mundane—food, bed linen, and dust mops—but billions went for more specifically medical equipment, from scalpels, syringes, and catheters to X-ray equipment, electronic blood cell counters, and artificial kidneys. In addition to the hospital market, physicians, dentists, nursing homes, and medical research labs spend huge sums, measured in the billions of dollars, on similar supplies.

The risks in the hospital supply industry appear to be as low as the profits are high. Medicaid may have its ups and downs, but Medicare, at least, is here to stay. And only a gambler with a compulsion for losing would bet against the likelihood of continued growth in hospital expenditures and increased subsidy of the market by the government. The hospital supply companies have gotten the message. "The start of IPCO's new financial year on July 1, 1966," said the 1967 annual report of IPCO, one of the major distributors and manufacturers of hospital goods, "also marked the beginning of the federal Medicare program and supplementary state health programs (Medicaid). The enormous increase in demand for institutional care . . . will, we believe, create a growing demand for the type of products IPCO distributes and manufactures." Like the man said, in the last dozen years IPCO's earnings have increased at a compound annual rate of twenty-two percent.

In the same vein, an executive of the paper manufacturer Kimberly-Clark, which has applied its technology to disposable bed linen and uniforms for hospitals, said, "The type of care usually provided under Medicare is the type that creates new opportunities for disposables." In 1951, $14 million worth of disposable products (including needles, syringes, and such standbys as paper plates) were sold. By 1965, the last pre-Medicare year, the market hit $100 million, and 1970 sales are expected to reach $300 million.

The stock market has been hot on the track. The month Medicare went into operation, stockbrokers Burnham and

Co. prepared an analysis of the industry for their customers. One year later, the Value Line Investment Survey (1966) spoke of one hospital supply company as "operating in a sector of the economy that is virtually recession-proof." (The company, American Hospital Supply, has seen its earnings grow at sixteen percent per year for the last decade. In the first half of 1969, earnings were up nineteen percent over the corresponding period of 1968.) And despite the Medicaid flip-flops, United Business Service listed eight hospital supply companies on its fall 1969 list of two hundred top growth stocks.

The traditional hospital supply companies—C.R. Bard, Becton-Dickinson, Baxter Labs, Sherwood Medical, Johnson and Johnson, IPCO, and American Hospital Supply—have been the big winners in the Medicare sweepstakes, with earnings up fifteen percent to twenty-five percent a year over the last few years. But the soaring profits and wide-open market are attracting new contenders as well. Through acquisitions of existing hospital supply companies or through applying the technology of other markets to medical supplies, many of the big guns of American industry are out for a piece of the pie. 3M Company is getting in through its mastery of cellophane—it makes peel-open packages of sterile surgical supplies, as well as surgical tapes and drapes and masks. Soap-maker Proctor and Gamble goes in for germicidal soaps and cleansers, rubber-maker B. F. Goodrich for antibacterial mattresses, and chemical company W. R. Grace for carbon dioxide absorbants for anesthesiology. Other big nonmedical companies buying in are, for instance, American Cyanamid and the Brunswick Corporation (a conglomerate). Companies with past experience in medical technology are especially active, with such big drug companies as Smith, Kline and French, Searle, Parke-Davis, Abbott, and Warner Lambert going into everything from blood bank equipment to cardiac pacemakers.

Supplies aren't the only thing booming in the hospital products industry. Medical electronics is moving out of the realm of science fiction and into the *Wall Street Journal.* A convergence of several factors has created a market currently running at about $350 million a year and expected to reach to one-and-a-half-billion dollars a year by the mid-1970s. For one thing, hospitals are buried under an increasing patient load. The volume of every service, from laundry to lab tests, from medical record-keeping to financial record-keeping, from diagnosis to intrahospital communications, is growing at a staggering rate. At the same time, the cost of the labor to perform these functions is rising sharply, under the impact of the hospital workers' unionization movement, newly applicable minimum-wage legislation, and an acute shortage of skilled medical manpower. The need of hospitals for cost-cutting technology has created a good sales pitch for the industry.

At the same time, years of government expenditures on defense and on medical research are flowering into a wealth of new technology to apply to hospitals. The new technology is expensive—out of the reach of the solo practitioner—but the large hospital has both the volume to use it effectively and the financial resources to afford it. And the costs can be passed along to the government in the form of Medicare and Medicaid depreciation allowances. "Medicare is the computer manufacturers's friend," exulted the trade journal Electronic News in April 1968.

Finally, at least some sectors of the electronics industry are under pressure to find new markets. The aerospace industry, for one, is in a trough, with NASA expenditures on the decline since 1965, Vietnam production past its 1968 peak, and a lag in new orders from the commercial airlines. Health—another government subsidized market—looks like a good pasture to head for.

One big chunk of the hospital electronic market is in computers. There are three types: general computers for business use like billing, accounting, payrolls; small machines built into other apparatuses, such as patient monitors; and computers for medical information and practice, including diagnosis, medical record-keeping, and "total hospital information systems". This last type of computer has not grown as rapidly as expected, due in part to the inherent irrationality of many hospital operations. Installation of a major computer must be preceded by a thorough systems-analysis of the hospital and rationalization of its procedures—often by experts supplied by the computer company. Most of the major computer companies are out for a share in the hospital market. They are joined by such outsiders as United Aircraft, Lockheed, Motorola, Xerox, and American Optical. Industry spokesmen estimate that upwards of a billion dollars worth of computers will have been installed in hospitals by 1975.

The general medical electronics industry is growing even more rapidly. Practically everybody who knows an oscilloscope from a stethoscope is out for this one—Litton Industries, G.E., International Rectifier, T.R.W., R.C.A., Varian, and Siemens, among the big ones. Perhaps the most intriguing product is produced by Fairchild Space and Defense Systems Division of Fairchild Camera and Instrument. It's a foreign body locator, patterned after mine detectors, for locating pieces of shrapnel bullets, or the safety-pin baby has swallowed. As with the parent electronics industry, a plethora of smaller companies like those lining Route 128 around Boston are appearing on the fringes. Hospital journals feature ads for such companies as Astro Associates, Spacelabs, Inc., Laser Systems and Electronics, Inc., and Medidata Services, Inc.

Like drugs in an earlier era, medical electronics has the potential to revolutionize medical practice. At one level, new vistas in diagnosis and treatment are opened up by the electron microscope, fiber optics, high energy radiation sources, computer analysis of electrocardiograms, and the like. At a second level, the potentials of computer diagnosis may lead to new roles for the doctor and other health workers. Finally, the need for systems-analysis to accompany the fully effective use of computers may have fallout in the form of partial rationalizations of hospital operations. But there is no guarantee that any of these changes will work to the favor of the patient. Like the drug companies' "me too" drugs, innovations may redound mainly to the favor of the manufacturers.

Health Insurance

The growth of private health insurance is superficially one of the great success stories of American business. In 1940, only twelve million Americans had the most common form of medical insurance, coverage for hospital expenses. By 1967, no less than 175 million, or eighty-three percent of the civilian population, were covered by private hospital insurance. One hundred million of these were covered by commercial, profit-making insurance companies, the rest by Blue Cross, Blue Shield, and independent plans. Many of these subscribers were insured for medical expenses other than hospitalization as well. The private companies collected premiums totaling $5.86 billion and paid out

$4.84 billion in benefits—administrative and selling expenses comprising much of the remainder.

Demand for health services has risen sharply since the early forties, just as the cost of those services skyrocketed beyond the reach of the average consumer. Some sort of insurance against the financial catastrophe of getting sick has become a necessity. Meanwhile, the forties and fifties saw the courts recognize fringe benefits as a legitimate area for collective bargaining, and mass purchasers of health insurance in the form of union and employer health-and-welfare-plans emerged. For these reasons, the health insurance industry grew explosively in the late 1940s and early 1950s. By now, more than one thousand companies, mainly life insurance companies, write health insurance. But the business is still dominated by a few giants: eight companies do almost two-thirds of the business.

The companies get a huge gross income from their health insurance business, but the profit picture is a bit muddy. Insurance companies earn money in two ways: directly, from premiums paid by consumers, and indirectly, from the investment of premiums in corporate and government securities. On the direct sale of health insurance to individuals, the companies generally make an underwriting profit. But on group policies, e.g., policies covering all the employees of a certain firm, the industry claims to lose money overall—about a quarter-billion dollars in 1967. And the investment income which the companies attribute to their health insurance business is, according to their claim, barely adequate to cover the underwriting loss.

Don't believe that the industry is writing health insurance for charity, though. Industry-wide, the companies may take an apparent underwriting loss, but most of the bigger companies report substantial and consistent profits. The losses probably reflect the trouble smaller companies have had in predicting expenses in the face of escalating medical prices. Industry giants, such as Equitable, Prudential, Metropolitan, have all showed net underwriting gains over the last five years. And the two big companies that did not, Aetna and Connecticut General, had one bad year that outweighed substantial gains in the other years.

The real profits in health insurance may be very different from the company claims. Insurance companies are good jugglers. Almost all companies link sales of health insurance to sales of life insurance, sometimes refusing to sell the one without the other. Thus the problems of allocating profits and costs between individual life, group life, individual health, group health, and various other kinds of policies are enough to turn an honest accountant's hair gray.

Finally, the insurance companies see health insurance, in the words of one insurance executive writing in the Health Insurance Review in April 1964, as "not so much a separate product but rather another of the client's needs." In many cases, health insurance is thrown in at a low price as a sweetener or loss leader for a highly profitable package including life insurance, disability, and even casualty insurance. The industry trade journals are full of such success stories as "Health Insurance—the Door Opener," and "Company Growth through Health Insurance."

For all these reasons, it is hard to say anything quantitative about the profits in the business. But health insurance is clearly an important component of the overall business of the life insurance companies. Health premiums alone account for fifteen to forty-five percent of the total gross income (including investments and all sorts of premiums) of the major companies. The entire life insurance industry had an after-tax income in 1967 of $9.1 billion, and had assets of $180 billion. The availability of such huge funds for investment makes control of the top companies a major source of corporate wealth and power. The health insurance business thus represents a significant piece of a very large pie indeed.

Despite its great size, the health insurance industry is about as functional as a dinosaur. Most Americans do have some kind of basic hospitalization insurance, but relatively few are covered for other medical expenses (forty percent for home or office physician visits, nine percent for nursing home care, two percent for dental expenses). Moreover, the insurance companies, along with their nonprofit buddy, Blue Cross, are caught in a cost squeeze: as prices for medical services rise, either the cost of insurance must go up or the expenses covered must be limited. Since commercial insurance companies set their premiums according to the medical experience of the individual group they are insuring, it is the elderly and other relatively high-risk persons who are squeezed out first.

The first consequence of the failures of commercial insurance came in 1965 when the companies were forced to relinquish older customers to Medicare. The companies' screams in response to Medicare had something of a theatrical quality. After all, the companies were ridding themselves of their least profitable customers. In fact, the year following Medicare saw a drop in company premiums but a much larger drop in benefit payments to consumers. But, as one company official told the *Wall Street Journal* in June 1965: "Most of us feel the loss of the over-65 market is not

the important thing, but rather what Medicare will do to
the business in ten or fifteen years." Industry executives
feared, according to the January 17, 1966 *New York Times*,
that "Medicare has brought the country a giant step
closer to socialized medicine" which could "all but eliminate the need for health insurance as it is sold today."
According to the *New York Times* article, the companies,
"generally inspired more by the wish to discourage government expansion of Medicare than by the desire for the
business that would be generated," cooperated with the
government in setting up the program. About fifteen companies now serve as intermediaries in the administration of
Medicare (see chapter VIII).

By 1968 it was again becoming evident that the health
insurance companies were not able to provide adequate
protection for many Americans. Under the influence of
problems affecting other aspects of the insurance business
and under pressure from consumer groups, the companies'
attitudes toward the government were shifting. Some industry figures openly hoped that the government would
serve as guarantor of the companies' market, rather than
as a competitor. One plan for national health insurance, for
instance, would have used government funds to subsidize
the purchase of private health insurance by employers and
employees. The president of Aetna was quoted in the July
1968 *Spectator* (an industry trade journal): "A program of
universal health insurance offers one way to spread the cost
of medicare [between employer, employee and govern-
ment]. It could be structured to retain the advantages of
competition and the profit incentive. . . . I have full confi-
dence in our ability to work successfully in partnership
with government."

Nursing Homes and Hospitals

The age-old way of profiting from illness is by selling health services themselves. Doctors have always done it; so have what are called proprietary (profit-making) hospitals and nursing homes. During all the fuss about the glamorous health hardware and electronics industries, old-fashioned health service profiteering hasn't been going out of style. If anything, nursing homes and hospital chains have become, at least to the adventurous investor, the hottest things going in the entire health industry, if not the entire stock market. Brokers and investment advisors liken the current boom in nursing homes and hospital chains to the boom in bowling alleys a few years ago or to that in computer software and fried chicken drive-ins today. In 1969 the nursing home industry, almost all of which is proprietary, grossed $2.8 billion, up twenty-one percent over 1968 and up 529 percent from 1960. Proprietary hospitals trailed with $720 million in total sales.

Only four years ago, the nursing home-and-hospital-business was still a cottage industry. A family added a wing to their home and called it a nursing home. A doctor or group of doctors bought and ran their own hospital for their own patients. Four years ago, only five nursing homes and one hospital company were publicly-owned, i.e., sold stock on the open market. Now there are fifty publicly-owned nursing home companies and six hospital companies.

What put the profit into the traditionally "charitable" nursing home and hospital business? Medicare, more than anything else, is underwriting the boom. The expansion of Blue Cross and commercial insurance coverage has helped, of course, to create hosts of paying customers for the health service business. Clever management is another factor. Nursing home and hospital companies are able to cut costs through economies of scale, such as bulk purchasing for an entire chain of facilities and centralized administration. But the voluntary (private, nonprofit) health sector also did much to set the stage for the entrance of the energetic profit-makers. Local voluntary hospital establishments, working with Blue Cross and regional health planning agencies, have done much to keep down the number of hospital and nursing home beds—creating a shortage which the profit-makers are eagerly filling.

Nursing homes are the ideal way to cash in on Medicare and Medicaid. Every oldster is at least partially covered and every oldster is a potential customer. Some of the largest publicly-owned nursing home companies are: Extendicare, Four Seasons Nursing Centers of America, Medicenters of America (a franchise system owned by Holiday Inns), and American Automated Vending Corporation. All are expanding; for instance, Four Seasons projects one hundred additional homes per year. Some buy existing homes; others build their own. Some operate their own homes; others are selling franchises.

If hotels are profitable, nursing homes ought to be profitable. But hospitals would seem to be another matter. Costs are wild; manpower is scarce and frequently irascible; funds are unreliable. To make a profit out of hospitals, you would have to forget all the old voluntary-sector inhibitions about hospitals as a sacred trust and a public service. This is exactly what the new hospital companies are doing: they select well-to-do neighborhoods and turn away any nonpaying patients who might find their way in. They avoid outpatient and emergency services insofar as possible. They encourage admission of short-term patients and reject those with chronic diseases in order to gain a high turnover rate (the first few days in the hospital pay the most). They avoid expensive and difficult technology, by concentrating on simple illnesses and elective surgery, and by contracting out for services such as pathology and radiology.

Wherever they spring up, profit-making hospitals offer stiff competition for the local voluntaries. First, they sell stock to local doctors, guaranteeing themselves a large medical staff and plenty of private patients. And of course the doctor stockholders have a special interest in keeping the hospital running efficiently and profitably. Once in operation, the profit-maker skims off the cream of the local patient crop from nearby voluntaries—the not-too-sick, able-to-pay patients. Having cut costs in all the ways listed above, the profit-maker is then able to lure nurses away from local voluntaries by offering higher salaries.

What's most insulting is for a profit-maker to parasitize off a local voluntary—setting up shop near a voluntary which can handle the newcomer's patient rejects and unprofitable services like obstetrics and outpatient care. This happened recently in Fort Meyers, Florida, where the Hospital Corporation of America (H.C.A.) decided to locate a new 150-bed profit-maker near the already underutilized voluntary Lee Memorial Hospital. When Lee Memorial protested against being left with the dregs of the patient supply, the H.C.A. president responded, "As proprietary hospitals we pay taxes. These taxes help support the tax-supported hospitals (voluntaries) which are in business to care for the nonpaying patient and were established for that purpose." Lee Memorial never intended to be quite *that* charitable, and is ganging up with the local power structure to drive out Nashville-based H.C.A. A recent *Fort Meyers News Press* editorial was entitled, "No Fast-Buck Hospital Needed Here."

If the hospital boom continues, it is likely to run into more and more organized opposition from voluntaries. Much of the opposition will be, on the surface at least, on moral grounds, although it is not clear why profits made by hospitals are any less moral than profits made by drug and hospital supply companies. But another element of the voluntary hospital leaders' opposition is probably pure snobbery: The men who head up the new hospital companies are not, by and large, the kind of men who would ever be chosen as trustees and directors of voluntaries. For example, American Medicorp, which does business primarily in the south and midwest, was founded by a couple of young Jewish lawyers from the north. The chairman and founder of H.C.A. is an ex-retail druggist who made his first fortune in the Kentucky Fried Chicken chain of drive-ins. To fight the profit-making intruders, voluntaries may have to swallow their traditional antipathy to government interference, and lobby for tougher laws regulating licensing and operation of hospitals.

In case government regulation is in the cards, many profit-making hospital companies are already one step ahead of the game—busily diversifying into hospital-related businesses. Beverly Enterprises, which owns eighteen hospitals and nursing homes, is forming Career Development Corporation, to train health personnel at a profit. Metrocare Enterprises, owner of nine acute-care hospitals, has purchased a construction firm and plans to build complete medical centers. Other companies are developing firms to provide ancillary services to hospitals. For instance, American Medical Enterprises, Inc. owns

Cardio-Pulmonary Services of America, Inc. (inhalation therapy); American Medicorp, Inc. has purchased Metropolitan Diagnostic Labs, Inc.

Coming from the other direction, a number of outside companies are diversifying into the profitable nursing home and hospital field. American Hospital Supply Corporation owns American Health Facilities, Inc., which constructs and furnishes nursing homes. Computer Research, Inc., runs Mental Retardation Centers, Inc.; and Cenco Instruments, Inc. has joined a nursing home consortium in Milwaukee.

The Health Industry Future

The health industry has come a long way from the days of the one-horse patent medicine peddler with his line of liver pills and elixirs. Replacing him are the mammoth internationalist drug companies, whose corporate medicine chests are increasingly likely to include hospital supplies, computers, and cosmetics along with a growing profusion of pills. Health insurance, which can trace its origins to pre-trade-union workers' welfare funds, is now a key element of the nation's vast insurance industry. The hospital supply industry has outgrown its bandaid days and is branching into catheters, computers, and artificial organs. Proprietaries, which used to be the dark horse of the delivery system, are forging multi-state chains and moving into more and more investors' portfolios. Two other components of the modern health industry bear watching: the hospital construction industry and the health systems consulting business. The health consultant of fifty years ago was likely to be the neighborhood barber; today the business includes defense-oriented think tanks like Rand, the Institute for

Defense Analysis, and Research Analysis Corporation.

The health industry has changed rapidly in the last five or ten years, that is, in the short period since the federal government has begun to play an important role in regulating and subsidizing health services and products. Changes in the future may be just as rapid and unpredictable, but two trends seem to be almost built in. First, the health industry will move increasingly into the mainstream of American industry. Corporate giants like Dow, DuPont, T.R.W. and Lockheed are busily staking out their claims on the profit-rich health turf. Drug companies, once the heavyweights of the health business, will be challenged by these newcomers. Secondly, the health industry will be pulling itself together into a more and more integrated monolith. The drug, hospital supply, and hospital equipment industries have already begun to blur into a single health products industry. Profit-making hospital chains are creating vertical chains including construction, supplies, and equipment. Insurance companies, so far aloof from the promiscuous merging in health products, may be about to take the plunge into direct provision of medical services, following the lead of nonprofit innovators like California's Kaiser plan and New York's Health Insurance Plan (HIP).

These developments in the health industry may have more impact on health services delivery than anything that happens in the next decade of medical research. What is emerging is an increasingly unified, significant sector of the U.S. economy with a major direct stake in the organization and financing of health services. In the past, drug companies dominated the health industry and they picked up their policy line from between the drug ads in the A.M.A. publications: up with solo, fee-for-service practice, down with government intervention of any sort. There's more to the health industry today than drugs, and many of the booming newcomers have market prospectives which reach far beyond the traditional, doctor-centered delivery system. And diversification into Medicare-subsidized, hospital-oriented products has seriously compromised the purity of the policy line of the drug companies.

It was Medicare that transformed the old bogeyman of government interference into a Santa Claus for the health industry. The drug industry and even the commercial insurance industry have found that they can live more than comfortably with Medicare and Medicaid. And of course it was Medicare that sent the hospital supply, equipment, and proprietary chain industries spiraling giddily into a boom. Within a few years the health industry may begin to outweigh organized consumer groups as the most powerful force lobbying for increased government subsidy for health services. The industry's interest, however, is in being subsidized with a minimum of regulation, as outlined, for instance, in some of the current proposals for a national health insurance. With national health insurance, the health industry could settle down to the kind of guaranteed security which the defense and aerospace industries enjoyed during the heyday of cold war spending.

When it comes to the health services delivery system, the health industry is again likely to line up with the medical liberals as opposed to the A.M.A. rear guard. Although only the proprietaries (hospitals and nursing homes) actually deliver services themselves, all segments of the health industry have an interest in increasing the productivity and efficiency of the delivery system. Insurance companies, which foot part of the bill, want to see health services become cheaper, or at least to see people utilize more of the cheaper services (e.g., clinic visits, as opposed to hospital stays). Drug, supply, and equipment dealers have an interest in increasing the total volume of health services delivered, since, for almost every provider-consumer encounter, a prescription is written, equipment is used, or a disposable is disposed of. This interest is not compatible with a fixation on solo physician practice—the least productive means for delivering health services. In fact, as far as the industry is concerned, there is no reason why the dispenser of drugs or the user of supplies and equipment should be a physician at all. The health industry may eventually join the ultraliberal faction of the medical world in advocating group practice and extensive use of paraprofessionals (if not machines) in direct patient contacts.

The hospital equipment industry has an even more immediate interest in the development of more centralized, institutionalized health services delivery systems. The market for heavy hardware such as computers, patient-monitoring devices and multi-phasic screening equipment is necessarily those health facilities which serve a large number of patients, rather than private offices. Furthermore, in order to absorb such equipment, health facilities must be moderately rational in their internal operations. (There's no point in getting a computer unless some of the hospital's operations are at least rational enough to program into it.) Looking beyond the individual facility, computer and electronics companies even have an interest in "rationality" at the regional level, i.e., in the development of multi-facility, regionally integrated health systems. The multi-hospital medical empire is the ideal market for computers to book admissions, for superspecialty hardware, and for TV systems to link outposts with centralized technical staff.

The danger in increasingly centralized, institutionalized

health delivery networks is, of course, that they will eventually get wise to the health products industry. Bulk buyers of pills, supplies and equipment could begin to exert significant leverage on prices and quality even before government regulation becomes a serious threat. However, if government subsidy of the health services delivery system is generous enough, hospitals will probably go on as they are now—hardly bothering to ask the price of pills and supplies. So long as the government is standing by to pick up the tab, the health industry's interest is in a delivery system which is boundlessly productive and mindlessly extravagant: organ transplants should be prescribed as frequently as tranquilizers are today, normal people should periodically have their blood cleaned out with an artificial kidney machine; "search and destroy" operations should become part of normal diagnostic work-ups.

To say that the health industry has an interest in a certain kind of delivery system is one thing; whether it can do anything about it is another question. So far the answer is yes—the health industry is developing increasingly effective ways of influencing public and private policy in health services delivery. At the most obvious level, the very existence of equipment which can be used only in hospitals, and of insurance which can be used only for hospital care, gives hospitals an edge over noninstitutional delivery modes. At the level of government policy, the health industry can always operate as an industry-wide lobby, testifying in Congressional hearings etc. Already, health industry people are beginning to show up regularly on important governmental panels and commissions. For instance, Nixon's top-level Taskforce on Medicaid and Related Programs includes a Director of Prudential Life Insurance Company. New York's 1967 Piel Commission, which was the launching pad for New York City's new Health and Hospitals Corporation (a quasi-public corporation set up to run the municipal hospitals) included the chairman of the board of the Systems Development Corporation, a leading consulting firm in health.

There are more direct and intimate ways in which the health industry influences and interacts with the delivery system. Trustees and upper-level staff of medical schools and hospitals are always welcome on the boards and top staffs of health industry firms and vice versa. Many hospital and medical school professionals moonlight as consultants to the health industry, thus acting as human bonds between the two worlds. Consulting in the other direction, industry to nonprofit delivery institutions, is more important in terms of volume and potential policy impact. For instance, Technomics Corporation, a consulting firm with links to the defense hardware industry, did much of the staff work for Mayor Lindsay's 1967 hospital commission (the Piel Commission). Another consultant, MacKinsey Corporation, is under contract to get the New York City Hospital Corporation off the ground. Interestingly enough, such consultants' recommendations invariably feature heavy use of computers and other expensive hardware. And as hospitals install more and more sophisticated systems, executives with backgrounds in health industry firms are increasingly moving into jobs in hospital administration.

No one seems to be too alarmed about the growing rapport between the health industry and the health services delivery system. On the contrary, it has become fashionable to look to the profit-motivated health industrial forces to lead the way out of the health services crisis. According to this view, what's been wrong with health services all along is that they've been isolated from the business world, cut off from the hard-headed management thinking, and of course, without the profit motive, unstimulated to really produce. But there is no reason yet to trust that the rationalizations that the health industry brings to health services will look like rationalizations to the consumer. Judging from America's experience with the drug industry, the consumer can expect no mercy from the new Medical-Industrial complex.

VIII

WHO PAYS THE PIPER . . .

From the consumers' point of view, there has been a health care crisis ever since American medical care grew out of drug store elixirs and hand-holding into a streamlined, space age commodity. Care has often been of low quality, usually unavailable when needed most, and always too expensive. But this crisis seemed to go on year after year, unnoticed except for occasional gripes, until recently. In 1969 something happened to make the health care crisis a matter of official national concern: medical costs rose so high so fast that it began to look as if health would soon be beyond the means of the richest nation on earth.

The cost of providing medical care—good, bad, or indifferent—has been the 1960s' Apollo mission of the consumer price index—up, up, and out of sight, (see chapter 9). While the overall cost of living climbed a complaint-worthy twenty-five percent over the last decade, the cost of a trip to the doctor climbed fifty percent—enough to make many a family put off trips to the doctor for minor illnesses, and general check-ups. Meanwhile, hospital costs doubled and then some. The basic room charge for a day in the hospital (not counting laboratory tests, medications, doctors' services, anesthesia, etc.) is close to $100 nationwide, and in some cities, $150 a day for a semiprivate room is not unheard of. The risk of serious illness has turned into a time bomb locked into the budget of the American middle-class family. Two weeks in the hospital can easily cost $5,000, wiping out the savings and repossessing the car of the average American family.

The high cost of providing medical care is not only a crisis for the consumer of care but for the provider, too. The hospital which runs up costs of $100 a day in elementary care for a patient has to get that $100 from somewhere, every day, or eventually it will have to close up shop. As costs get so high that an increasing number of patients cannot possibly pay their bills themselves, the hospitals must hope that their patients will have insurance, or that government programs will pay for their care. But many patients can't even afford insurance premiums (which are of course ultimately based on the costs of the benefits offered). And government and the insurance companies are increasingly using their bargaining power to avoid paying the full costs of care. The result is instant crisis—exactly what happened in 1969. In New York, fifteen voluntary (nonprofit) hospitals threatened to shut down complaining that Medicaid was not paying the full bill of their patients and that many other patients who were too rich to be eligible for Medicaid were welshing on their bills. In Philadelphia, several leading private hospitals came close to closing their emergency rooms in the summer of 1969. Articles began to appear with increasing frequency on the crisis in American medicine. And for the first time in two decades, significant business, labor, and medical forces began to line up behind demands for a national health insurance program.

If the crisis in the financing and delivery of medical care seems to have appeared suddenly, it is because over the last three decades, we have been rescued by one makeshift solution after another. Back in the golden twenties, rich philanthropists underwrote the costs of most voluntary (private, nonprofit) hospitals. These charitable subsidies helped keep the cost down for the user of services. But philanthropy went down the drain with the stock market in 1929, and never recovered. Hospital costs were, of course, much cheaper in those days. But patients were much poorer, too, and, as patients failed to pay their bills, hospitals saw their income shrink more rapidly than their costs. The hospitals soon found (or rather invented) a new "third party" to pay the bill (the patients and the providers of service are considered the first and second parties)— Blue Cross and Blue Shield. Blue Cross (see chapter X) emerged out of a 1929 arrangement between the school teachers of Dallas, Texas, and Baylor University Hospital. The hospital had noticed that the unpaid bills of school teachers weighed heavily on their ledgers. They therefore proposed that teachers pay the hospital a small, manageable, monthly fee. In return, the hospital guaranteed the teachers up to twenty-one days free use of a semiprivate room and other hospital services. For the teachers, the fear of being wiped out by a high hospital bill was gone; for Baylor, the problem of uncertain income from the teachers' use of the hospital was solved. This first "Blue Cross" plan had several characteristics which were to become the pattern for other such plans: the plan provided service benefits (i.e., so many days in the hospital regardless of actual costs) rather than a cash indemnity. And the plan was not managed by some impersonal outside concern— it was sponsored and largely controlled by the hospitals.

Similar plans rapidly appeared elsewhere. The next step in complexity was to extend the program to all the hospitals in an area. The subscriber thus paid a monthly fee to a central agency, Blue Cross, set up by the participating hospitals. In return, the plan paid for the cost of the subscriber's stay in whichever hospital he used, up to a certain limit. As the movement toward such plans spread, the national association of voluntary hospitals—the American Hospital Association—offered the use of the trademark "Blue Cross" to any such plan which met Association standards. State legislatures pitched in and made the plans tax-exempt, freed them from certain provisions of the state insurance laws, and subjected them to loose state regulation.

Blue Cross covered only the cost of hospitalization perse. It was left to Blue Shield to cover medical and surgical expenses inside the hospital (neither plan covers out-of-hospital care). Like Blue Cross, Blue Shield was a child of the Depression, born of the doctor's needs to protect his income. Behind Blue Shield were the medical societies (or local doctors' guilds) rather than the hospitals. They were motivated, however, more by the threat of government intrusion into medical care insurance—an ever-vivid fear to the A.M.A.—than by a commitment to provide comprehensive services. In the words of medical economists Anne and Herman Somers, Blue Shield had a "defensive coloration." As a result, its benefits have always been more limited than those of its companion Blue Cross.

Both Blues grew rapidly. From a half million subscribers in 1935, Blue Cross's membership hit six million in 1940, thirty-seven million in 1950, and some sixty-eight million by 1969. (In addition, about six million over-sixty-five-year-old Americans have Blue Cross coverage supplementary to their federal Medicare benefits). Compared to Blue Cross, Blue Shield has been slow to bloom. Blue Shield's surgical insurance covered only 260 thousand people as late as 1940, and has grown to about sixty million at present.

The next third parties to appear on the scene were the commercial, profit-making insurance companies—Metropolitan, Equitable, Aetna, etc. (see chapter VII). Commercial health insurance, although it has a history reaching back to the late nineteenth century, is basically a postwar phenomenon. After the war, with burgeoning trade unions ready to bargain with employers for mass life and health insurance policies for their members, the insurance market cracked wide open. Especially in the medical-surgical fields, which were only partially and grudgingly covered by Blue Shield, the commercials saw open daylight. By 1969, commercial health insurance companies had the bulk of the business, with some one hundred million subscribers (both individuals and members of group plans) buying hospital insurance, and almost as many people buying surgical insurance.

In most states, however, the Blues still remain the single dominant force in the health insurance field, since the commercial business is divided up among some ten or so major companies and hundreds of smaller ones. The Blue Cross hegemony over health policy has been strengthened by its intimate relationship to the hospitals. It is Blue Cross which has been continually concerned with policy issues in the delivery of health care; the commercial companies have until recently paid little attention to these matters and have concerned themselves purely with paying bills.

By the late 1950s, as health costs began their relentless rise, it became clear that the private insurance mechanisms, the Blues and commercials, were hopelessly inadequate. There were, from the consumers' point of view, many medical services still not covered by insurance. And there were still many people who could not afford insurance at all—the poor and the elderly (who overlap considerably). To make matters worse, these people tended to use more medical care than the average citizen and were thus quoted higher rates for insurance. The result: those who needed health care (and health insurance) most were least able to pay for it. This posed problems from the hospitals' point of view, too, since these patients, in emergencies at least, still used health services, but were unable to pay for them. The more costs rose, the worse the problem became. We seemed to be back in the thirties again but with all the prices doubled.

After several years of debate, the federal government decided to step into the third party game to solve the problem. In 1965, Medicare and Medicaid were enacted into law. Medicare was a government-operated insurance program for the elderly. Like conventional insurance, the insured had to pay premiums, in the form of payroll taxes. Added to the revenue from payroll taxes was a hefty government subsidy so that the total amounted to more or less adequate insurance for those over sixty-five. Medicaid (see chapter XI) worked on very different principles. Under Medicaid, the federal government provided matching grants to states and local governments, financed out of general tax revenues, to pay directly for the health services used by certain categories of the poor. In both cases, however, the government was simply acting as a third party, for the poor in one case and for the aged in the other. The poor and the aged received health care; the hospitals and doctors who treated them got their bills paid. At present, some twenty million people are covered under Medicare; and some eleven million under Medicaid.

Forty years after the first Blue Cross plan got going, third party payments are now the life blood of the American medical economy. In a typical big city voluntary hospital upwards of ninety percent of patients' bills are paid by one or another of the third parties (Blue Cross, Medicaid, Medicare, commercial insurance companies). These various sources thus provide a more or less stable income which is very close to the entire operating financial needs of the institutions. They provide the funds for raising the wages of low-paid orderlies and nurses' aides and for operating the increasingly complex equipment which is a part of modern medical care. They pay the salaries of forty-thousand-dollar-a-year hospital directors and provide the profit margins for the multi-billion dollar hospital supplies industry. In short, they are the financial base upon which the entire American hospital system, and, increasingly, the entire American health care system rests.

How then can the hospitals and the consumers still face a crisis situation? The answer would have sounded like blasphemy only a couple of years ago: the very third party mechanisms which for so long were thought to be the solution to the ills of the American health care system have turned out to be one of the greatest problems. They are at one and the same time the major cause of the runaway costs of the medical system, and a major institutional source of power defending the status quo and preventing major reorganizations of the medical care system from occurring.

The third party payment agencies have boosted costs through the very mechanism by which they (especially Blue Cross, Medicare, and Medicaid) pay the hospitals for services. Ever since the hospitals set up the first Blue Cross to ensure that their bills were paid (not to ensure that patients got service) each of these third parties has paid the hospitals whatever the hospital claims is the actual cost of providing services. For the hospitals, this has meant that third parties do not merely provide a stable income; they are a perpetual Santa Claus. Whatever the hospital wants by way of fancy new equipment, luxury accommodations, high-priced doctors, or administrators (or even public relations men or full-time lobbyists), the third party will pay for. A cost-plus contract, whether in the defense industry or in the hospital business, provides no incentives for saving money. There is no reason to be efficient, to purchase new equipment only if needed, to provide the maximum amount of care for the dollar. The "cost pass-through" provided by third party payments has allowed the hospitals (and, to a lesser extent, other providers of medical care) to be financially entirely irresponsible, and it is this, more than anything else, that has sent the cost of health care skyrocketing. All through the forties and fifties, the years of Blue Cross domination, health care costs rose steadily at a more rapid pace than costs of other consumer goods and services. Then, in 1965, the biggest chunk yet of third party financing arrived, all in a single dose (Medicare and Medicaid). The lid on hospital spending went flying off. The results show up most clearly in the hospital supplies industry. Profits of leading companies doubled in four years, and stock brokers rhapsodized over the stocks of such outfits as American Hospital Supply.

With all this largesse, then, how can the hospitals scream that they are underfinanced? Most of the hospitals' complaints come from the fact that the government, horrified at the Pandora's box they opened with Medicaid and Medicare, has tried to cut back on both programs. Meanwhile, in the face of rising health care costs, the cost of private health insurance has soared, too. As a result, an increasing number of people fall into no man's land—too rich for Medicaid, too young for Medicare, too poor to buy private health insurance, and certainly too poor to pay hospital bills. At the same time, the third parties, in a desperate attempt to keep their own costs down, are tightening up on their reimbursement formulas, scrutinizing bills more carefully for unnecessary expenditures, and so forth.

The result is that once again hospitals, hospital supply companies, businesses, unions, governments are looking again to the solution which has so often before gotten them out of this jam—find a new third party mechanism. But the lessons of the past are that if you leave any group of people out of the third party system, they rise up to haunt you by not paying their bills. So this time the solution advanced is "universal" (or "national") health insurance, subsidized by the government (see chapter XII). There is only one difficulty: Blue Cross and the private insurance companies already exist. They aren't about to have the government come and cut them out of the action. And their powerful allies among the hospitals and the companies that supply the hospitals fear that a government program would bring closer scrutiny and an end to the glory days of unrestricted costs-plus payments. So they, too, want to preserve the old generous third party mechanisms, working them somehow into a government-subsidized insurance system.

Patients, who want only decent, available health care, may not care about preserving Blue Cross or letting the hospital directors and doctors spend freely. But patients will have very little to say about the next jury-rigged solution to the financing crisis.

IX

THE PRICES GO UP, UP, UP

August 1969. John DeLury, president of New York City's Sanitationmen's Union, told a state hearing on a proposed rate increase for Blue Cross about the hospitalization of the son of one of his members: "A ten year old boy was admitted to a hospital at 3:20 A.M. The boy died at 10:34 the same night. The family of this child was charged $105.80 for drugs, $184.80 for X-rays, $220.00 for inhalation therapy, $655.50 for laboratory work. The total bill for the child was $1,717.80, or $86.73 per hour of hospitalization."

Another union man was hospitalized for sixty days. His total bill was $22,147.95, an average of $369.13 a day. The union welfare plan called in a doctor to review the bill. Said the doctor: "I am struck by the fact that while charges for daily care (room and board) averaged $52.00 daily, the charges for medication and laboratory tests amounted to twice those of daily care [averaging $104.27 and $102.58 daily, respectively]. During these sixty days, he was subjected to more than 1100 laboratory tests, transfusions, and medications. I do not challenge the indications for such a heroic form of therapy, but am forced to conclude that few humans can survive such intensive care."

August 1969. Thirteen nonprofit hospitals in New York City announced that they were in "desperate" financial straits—on the verge of closing. The source of their trou-

bles? Rising costs of providing hospital services had out-
run any available means of paying these costs.

September 1969. A wave of requests by Blue Cross for rate
increases swept the country—25 percent in Connecticut,
50 percent in New York, 33 percent in Rhode Island, 44
percent in New Jersey. As a result of the 43 percent rate
hike finally granted in New York, some families will pay
as much as $108 a year more for their hospitalization insur-
ance. Blue Cross' explanation of the increase? The rates
the insurance organization had to pay hospitals for their
subscribers' hospital stays had soared.

August 1969. Leon J. Davis, president of the union representing workers in New York City voluntary hospitals,
threatened a New York State legislative committee investigating Medicaid with "the biggest crisis this city has ever
seen" if a new state law designed to hold down hospital
costs were put into effect. Davis denounced the law as
"little more than a freeze on the wages of people who work
in hospitals."

"No other workers' wages are being controlled," union
representatives elaborated at a hearing of the New York
Mayor's Committee on Inflation, a few months later.
"There are no controls on doctors' fees or the profits of the
drug companies and hospital supply companies who make
billions in profits off of sick people."

You don't have to read the newspapers to know that the
costs of health care are soaring. Anyone who has used, is
using, or considering using hospitals and clinics knows
that hospital costs are rising even faster than the price of
a sirloin steak. New York paced the pack. The cost of a day
in the hospital in the New York area went up sixteen
percent in 1968, thirteen percent in the first seven months
of 1969 alone. Prestige hospitals, like New York Hospital

and Presbyterian, charge up to $140 or $150 a day for a semiprivate room, and it's hard to find a hospital room anywhere in the city for less than $80 a day. Other cities are not far behind. Nationwide, the cost of a day in the hospital has doubled since 1962.

At these prices, even a middle-class family can have their life savings wiped out by a single illness. As a result, families must buy insurance against illness, through "nonprofit" systems such us Blue Cross or through commercial companies. But now even hospital insurance rates are soaring out of people's reach. New York Blue Cross, which covers more than eight million people, now charges families rates as high as $312 a year—for benefits which are shrinking as fast as hospital costs are rising (see chapter X).

When it comes to purchasing health care, most people have no choice—they have to get it, whatever the price. Not so with the government, which pays for more than a third of the nation's hospital care through programs like Medicare and Medicaid and through direct operation of municipal, state and federal hospitals. Hospital costs have been rising rapidly for years, but when they began to skyrocket out of sight two years ago, New York State chopped more than a million people off the Medicaid rolls in New York City alone. The same story has been repeated throughout the nation. In effect, the state was saying that it couldn't pay the high-cost hospital bills any longer, that people would just have to fend for themselves. Yet those cut off Medicaid certainly can't afford hospital costs any better than the state can. When illness strikes, these people will have to fall back on municipal hospitals, or voluntary hospitals' charity wards.

In turn, these institutions have said, "We can't cope with rising costs, either." One after another, they have shut

their doors to the poor, e.g., voluntary hospitals have ger-
rymandered their service areas to exclude low-income
areas and have cut down their clinic services. Meanwhile,
the municipal and county hospitals are fiscally and physically in no shape to pick up the patient load as the private
hospitals cut down on services.

It's a vicious cycle: hospital costs rise so rapidly that
everyone has to have some kind of insurance in case of
illness. At the same time, the insurance becomes more
expensive (like Blue Cross) or less available (like Medicaid). For more and more people, middle-class as well as
poor, health care is not a right, and not even a privilege—
as the A.M.A. would have it—but a luxury.

When costs go up, a lot of people get hurt. At the same
time, the dollars of increased costs have to go somewhere.
According to New York Blue Cross, between 1964 and
1969 the cost of a day in a local hospital went up eighty-four
percent. Hospital service did not improve any eighty-four
percent during that time. Where, then, did the money go?

Hospital officials' answers are as evasive as they are infre-
quent. One spokesman for the voluntary hospitals said on
CBS radio in late 1969 that operating a hospital is "a sacred
trust" and not something that can be measured in dollars
and cents. Another spokesman, Monsignor James H. Fitz-
patrick, president of the Greater New York Hospital Association and executive director of Catholic Medical Center
of Queens and Brooklyn, explained at the 1969 hearings
into Blue Cross' rate hike request that the additional
money is used "for one thing and one thing only—to re-
lieve human suffering, to treat, and, if possible, to cure
disease, above all, to save human life."

Other hospital administrators deny that there is anything amiss in high hospital costs. Martin Steinberg, then

director of Mount Sinai Hospital in New York, suggested to his fellow hospital administrators that they not be so apologetic about costs. In an article in the January, 1968, *Journal of the American Hospital Association* dramatically entitled "Hospital Costs are Much Too Low," Steinberg comments: "Our attitude has been altogether too defensive. We seem to be sharing in the horror of the public spokesmen about the high and ascending level of costs. . . . The public will have to understand that the cost of the war against disease can only be limited by the nature of the enemy, and that if we are to win, if we are to be a healthy people, the necessary armaments and measures must be paid for."

The cost line cannot be held, according to this school. To impose "desperate economies" on the hospitals, Yonkers (New York) General Hospital administrator Clarence W. Duryea told the Blue Cross rate increase hearing, "is to play a dangerous game with the lives and well-being of the patients who now look to us for the care they need." The only way out of the never-ending cost increases, says Duryea, is "either closing the doors of our institutions to some or all of our patients, or else short-changing them by deliberately lowering the quality of care we provide."

Pinned down, the hospitals blame the cost rise on two main factors. First, labor costs have soared, and, since about two-thirds of the cost of running a hospital consists of salaries and fringe benefits for employees, this has boosted costs. Second, you get more for your day in the hospital today than yesterday—more lab tests, more treatment procedures, more artificial kidneys, more radiation therapy, etc. "Expensive?" say the Blue Cross radio and TV ads, "But it's worth it."

These explanations are related to the facts, but only

distantly. First, the matter of hospital costs: salary costs in short term nongovernmental hospitals in the New York area rose ninety-six percent in the last five years, according to Blue Cross (about fifteen percent more rapidly than in the nation as a whole). Part of this represented the wages of the additional employees needed to care for a growing patient load. Between half and two-thirds of the remaining increase (i.e., of the increased labor costs per patient-day) reflected higher wages for people who work in hospitals; the rest stemmed from a rise in the number of employees required to care for a single patient. (The latter is in part a result of shorter hours for employees, in part a reflection of the greater complexity of care.)

But the increase in hospital labor costs requires closer examination. First of all, hospital workers' wages were historically extremely low, and remain low. As recently as ten years ago, unskilled workers in major New York City hospitals received twenty-eight to thirty dollars a week for forty-four to forty-eight hours of work. Many full-time hospital workers were on welfare. Hospital costs were thus actually higher than they appeared, but part of the cost was paid through taxes for the welfare system. In effect, the great philanthropic institutions were supported primarily through the philanthropy not of their rich benefactors but of their poor employees, who donated their labor to keep the hospitals going. Wages have crept up since that time. In New York City, where most unskilled and semiskilled hospital workers are now unionized, present contracts call for minimum wages of $100 a week (in the voluntary hospitals), and the average wage for unionized employees (which excludes registered nurses, doctors, supervisors, and administrators) is estimated by union organizers at about $120 a week. This is still $2500 less than the median

family income in New York City, and is about $5000 less
than the U.S. Bureau of Labor Statistics estimate for a
"moderate" standard of living for a family of four in the
city.

Outside of New York City and a few other unionized
areas, the picture is much bleaker. In late 1968, union and
management officials estimated that nonprofessional hospital workers in Syracuse averaged less than seventy dollars a week. And until the appearance of union organizers
in the late spring of 1969, minimum hospital wages in
cities such as Philadelphia and Baltimore were $1.60 an
hour.

Second, the ninety-six percent increase in salary expense can by no means by entirely attributed to employees
in the categories represented by unions. The wages of all
kinds of hospital employees have risen dramatically. While
orderlies' wages went from sixty or seventy dollars a week
to $100 a week in New York over the last four years, the
average net incomes of full-time hospital radiologists' were
jumping from $26,000 to about $34,000. Interns and residents, formerly poorly paid, now receive $9,000-$11,000 a
year. Senior hospital physicians get salaries of $40,000 and
up, and often find plenty of time for a lucrative private
practice on the side. Hospital administrators are also in on
the salary splurge. New York's Lenox Hill Hospital is
reported to have recently offered City Hospital Commissioner Joe Terenzio their top administrative post at a salary
of $75,000 a year, and the median income for top hospital
chief executives has been estimated at over $40,000. About
twenty-five to thirty-five percent of hospital employees are
in categories such as physician, administrator, or supervi-
sor, and since these are generally the higher paid positions,
a considerably larger proportion of the hospitals' salary

expense presumably goes to keep these hospital workers in high income brackets.

In their haste to blame their workers for forcing costs up, the hospitals usually fail to note that nonlabor costs have risen just as rapidly as labor costs, nationwide. In New York, according to Blue Cross, nonsalary expenses in voluntary hospitals rose sixty-three percent between 1964 and 1969. (This figure actually underestimates the costs attributable to increased expenditures on goods and services. For example, a major component of increased labor costs is the increased number of employees required to operate all the new computers, diagnostic equipment, etc., that hospitals have recently purchased.) Part of this rise, according to the hospitals, is from the economy-wide inflation. Food, linen, and other budget items all cost more. But mainly, say the hospitals, the cost rise comes from the greater complexity of present methods of treatment. For example, in 1963, only eighteen percent of all community hospitals had intensive care units; by 1968, forty-two percent had installed and were operating such units. Similar statistics hold for such expensive miracles as hyperbaric chambers, open heart surgery units, renal dialysis programs, and extensive diagnostic testing programs.

Stockbrokers also enthuse about these miracles (see chapter VII). Hospital supplies and medical electronics are the glamor stocks of 1969-70. In past years, drugs, another product dispensed by hospitals, have been the most profitable business in America. Now hospital supply companies, with profits growing at a rate of more than twenty percent a year, are nudging their pharmaceutical companions.

Hospital managers and stockbrokers may glow over the new medical miracles, but patients are entitled to some doubts. First, there is reason to doubt the judgment of the hospitals about the great importance of these items to the overall health of people. As is the case with drugs, most of the information about them comes from the companies which produce them. The buyer of the new medical technology does not generally have the specialized knowledge or the time to evaluate the product or to figure out how much it should cost him. With literally hundreds of companies competing for a share of the market for such devices as electrocardiographs, defibrillators, and patient monitors, the average hospital administrator or the average physician is in no position to determine whether a particular feature of one model which adds several hundred or thousand dollars to the cost is really important or whether it is merely the medical electronics equivalent of a chromium tail-fin.

Second, there is no reason to think that the hospitals are particularly concerned about the cost of the devices they buy. In the final analysis, the hospitals don't pay the bill, anyhow. The consumer pays, directly or through a third party—Blue Cross, Medicaid, or another. But the third party payment mechanisms are the hospital world's version of the cost-plus contract used by the Defense Department to reward its contractors. The insurers pay the hospitals whatever the hospital claims was its actual cost of providing service. If the hospital buys and operates a computer, or an intensive care unit, the cost of providing a day's services rises. Automatically, the rate at which Blue Cross, Medicare, and Medicaid reimburse the hospitals also rises. It makes no difference whether the computer or the high energy radiation unit was really necessary, whether it was overpriced, misused, or whether it adds significantly to the overall quality of health care the hospital can deliver. The hospital has no reason, therefore, to be careful how it spends its money—it gets paid in any case.

One result of the irresponsibility this permits is the unnecessary duplication of equipment and faciities. Hospitals compete to buy the prestigious pieces of equipment which fit into the physicians' research programs and the trustees' ego trips. For example according to Montefiore (New York) Hospital Director Martin Cherkasky in a testimony to a 1969 Senate hearing (himself one of the big purchasers of hospital equipment in the city): "We have fifteen open heart programs in the city of New York. Seven of those open heart programs do eighty-three percent of all the heart surgery; eight of them do seventeen percent. Those eight who do seventeen percent do about one case a month. Do you know what it costs to maintain the specialized equipment and the specialized personnel when you do one case a month? . . . Not only is it expensive, but the quality is miserable, since only a cardiac surgical team constantly at work can produce the quality care that is needed."

Third, what a hospital considers a necessary expenditure may not be the expenditure which would maximally benefit the public health. Hospitals have other priorities—research, education, and prestige—which may compete with community health needs. For example, a few years ago Mount Sinai Hospital in New York City installed a three-quarter-million-dollar hyperbaric chamber—the only one in New York. The chamber costs more than $600,000 a year to operate. In its five years of operation it has been used for some 450 major operations and some 400 treatments for other medical conditions that benefit from high-pressure oxygenation—that is, about 190 times a year in all. The chamber may be a life saver for some (although some doctors have recently expressed doubts about its value to any patients), but for the same cost, Mount Sinai could deliver 20,000 outpatient visits a year, or set up a vast program to screen children in surrounding East Harlem for lead poisoning and anemia. But it is the hospital that chooses how to allocate its spending, not the community. And so, the cost of hospital care goes up, but health care is not, on balance, necessarily maximally improved.

Expensive hardware, no matter how redundant, usually benefits *someone.* An incalculable portion of hospital costs, however, is of no direct benefit to the patients and sometimes represents sheer waste. For instance, it is widely acknowledged that hospitals are often inefficiently run. Two years ago, a study by the National Advisory Commission on Health Manpower indicated that *per diem* costs in twelve "distinguished" hospitals, comparable in terms of services performed, teaching functions, quality of staff etc., varied from $46 to $96 a day after correction for differing wage rates. Similar variations occurred in all the components of total cost—dietary, housekeeping, nursing, administration. One can only conclude that hospitals vary greatly in efficiency, i.e., that some hospitals are just plain wasteful. One hospital administrator, Donald C. Carner of Memorial Hospital in Long Beach, California, has estimated that improved purchasing and personnel practices, better utilization of technology, less duplication of resources, and improved utilization of presently employed manpower could lead to savings averaging about ten to fifteen percent of total costs.

Many hospital expenditures are not even nominally for providing services to patients. The best publicized expenses in this category are those for research and for the education of medical students, interns and residents, and nurses. These costs are partially covered by government grants, student tuition payments, and the like. But a hefty chunk is left over. Hospitals seek to cover the deficit through charges to patients. (Blue Cross Medicaid and Medicare refuse to pay these costs unless they are directly related to the care of patients. In other words, if you show a resident how to perform a procedure on a patient, it's paid for by Blue Cross; if you give him a lecture in a classroom, it's not.)

The question is not whether or not research and education are important. A rational and humane society would certainly devote sizeable resources to them. The question is whether or not the research and education we are getting are worth the price. Is a ghetto-based big city hospital the place for research on basic genetic mechanisms in viruses—research which, at best, holds only a distant promise for medical care? Should a hospital charge its patients for investigation on a rare, neurological disease, when basic preventive care is unavailable in the neighboring community? Should it train a few hundred Ivy Leaguers to be Park Avenue specialists? Or should it use its vaunted facilities and staff to develop programs to train black or Puerto Rican youngsters, whose academic background is not up to Harvard standards, to become highly competent doctors serving their community? At present, it is the doctors and the hospitals who decide, without any accountability to the public, what research shall be done, who shall be trained, and how. But it is the person who happens to be sick at any given time who foots the bill.

Another form of hospital expenditure, which is totally unrelated to patient care, is bank interest. In the past, major capital expenditures (expenditures for buildings and major equipment) by hospitals were financed primarily through philanthropy and the government's Hill-Burton program. But nowadays hospitals are more and more likely to use their own operations to generate capital funds. They save their profits; even a nonprofit hospital may have income in excess of expenditures. They hoard the depreciation allowance included in third party reimbursements. And increasingly, they borrow from banks, paying off the loans out of charges to their patients.

In 1969, the year of the hospital crisis, many hospitals started turning to the banks for operating funds as well as for capital funds. One grim week in October, New York's prestigious Albert Einstein College of Medicine is said to have been forced to borrow to meet its payroll, and another New York City hospital had to ask First National City Bank to grant it a one-year moratorium on repayments of a $350,000 loan.

Of course, at current high interest rates, the banks are making quite a pile off the hospitals. One New York hospital is currently paying $1.25 million a year in mortgage and other interest. That figures out to about three dollars a day of every patient's bill going right into the bank's profit ledgers.

In addition to research and education and interest—expenditures which have some relation however distant at times, to a hospital's patient care mission—hospitals spend money for purposes which are in no way related to the welfare of their patients. They hire public relations specialists at $20,000 a year and up to clean up their image with a public which is increasingly disenchanted with the angels of mercy. They spend hundreds of thousands of dollars in efforts to prevent their employees from organizing themselves into unions. They furnish their directors' offices in Danish modern, their lobbies in wall-to-wall carpet, and their entrances in patio-to-roof marble.

Why, then, are hospitals expensive? In part, because of rising (but still low) wages for nonsupervisory employees. In part, because good medical care is increasingly complex. But hospitals are also expensive because they have become outlets for the greed and ambition of some of the most profitable private businesses and some of the most grasping private businessmen in the United States—drug and hospital supply companies, physicians, and hospital administrators. Hospitals are expensive because these men and companies have uncontested control over the spending of the dollars of taxpayers and patients—a control which they exercise arrogantly, inefficiently, and with little concern for the health needs of the community. From an economic point of view, hospitals are on their way to being little more than conduits, places where consumer and taxpayer money is funneled into private profits. If the helter-skelter pace is too great and forces a few hospitals in low-income areas to close, so what? Hospitals these days aren't run for charity.

Meanwhile, high hospital costs have become a good excuse for cutting back on Medicaid and limiting non-self-supporting community care. And the hospitals and the government are trying to rouse up the anger of the community against the hospital workers who by their wage demands have supposedly forced up hospital costs. When someone profits, someone else loses. The people who lose on the hospitals' business are hospital workers and the people who need hospital care.

X

THE BLUE CROSS WE BEAR

All over the country, people are increasingly cross at Blue Cross. In other states around the nation, headlines have announced massive rate increases for the hospital-insurance organization: forty-three percent in New York, twenty-five percent in Connecticut, forty-four percent in New Jersey, thirty-three percent in Rhode Island, other huge boosts in Massachusetts, Maryland, and upstate New York. Despite outraged opposition from labor groups, civic organizations, local governments, and just about everyone else who could remotely be considered a consumer, the rate increases rolled onward and upward.

Confronted with a national crisis in medical costs, Blue Cross pleads not guilty. It argues that it is merely the collection agency for the hospitals, raking off only a subsistence level overhead for itself. But hospital costs are not rising like the price of bread or clothing—they are rising at three times the rate of the Consumer Price Index. There is something gravely wrong with the American health system. And, at the center of that system—paying the bills, planning new programs, manipulating both public and private health policy—is Blue Cross. With the exception of the American Medical Association, no single agency, public or private, has ever had such a grip on American health policy.

Blue Cross is the central mechanism for financing hospital care in America. The entire structure of the hospital system—its finances, its manpower policies, and often even its medical policies—rests upon Blue Cross as a base. Blue Cross insures the hospitals that they will have a reasonably stable income. It ensures the hospital-supply companies and drug companies of a stable market. It insures the urban medical schools and their affiliated hospitals that their research and training priorities will not be challenged by their sources of financing.

There are seventy-five Blue Cross plans in the United States. Each plan is independent, providing hospitalization insurance in a certain geographical area, usually a state or city. The Blues are nonprofit, tax-exempt organizations. They are usually set up under special state legislation which exempts them from certain provisions of the state insurance laws but which subjects them to regulation by a state agency, often the state insurance department. The plans are linked by the national Blue Cross Association, which represents them in national affairs, provides services in marketing, education, research, and professional and public relations, and operates an interplan bank which provides coverage for Blue Cross subscribers using hospital benefits outside the area of their own plan. Together, the Blue Cross plans provide hospitalization insurance for sixty-eight million Americans, as well as insurance supplementary to Medicare for another six million people over age sixty-five. Almost seven billion dollars a year passes through Blue Cross. (Blue Cross pays only hospital bills; doctors' bills, even in the hospital, are covered separately by Blue Cross' companion organization, Blue Shield.)

Blue Cross is a powerful community force. Its trustees sit on business, university, and hospital boards. Blue Cross officers sit on local, state, and federal government councils on health issues. Blue Cross thus has the position and the power to play a major role in coordinating the health interests of these various sectors. In this role, as we shall see it acts as the collective representative of the long-term interests of the hospitals.

The operations of Blue Cross are not limited to its role as the largest private financier of hospital care. The plans also provide most of the machinery for operating the Medicare and Medicaid programs—they act as intermediaries between the government and most hospitals. Although the government ultimately pays the bill for medical services offered under Medicare and Medicaid, it does not ordinarily pay the hospitals directly. Rather it funds the intermediary—usually Blue Cross—which in turn pays the hospital. The exact rate of payment is negotiated between the hospitals and the intermediary. This puts Blue Cross in a key position to determine how the federal programs are run. One measure of Blue Cross' importance to these programs is that more than ninety percent of the hospitals' Medicare bills are paid through Blue Cross. In eighteen states, Blue Cross is also the intermediary through which Medicaid bills are paid. Federal programs account for almost half of Blue Cross' operations: the number of Blue Cross employees has doubled since the birth of Medicare.

Blue Cross has its eyes out for any further expansion of government's role in financing health care. For example, President Nixon has opposed any government-financed national health insurance scheme ever since, as a freshman congressman, he fought against President Truman's proposals. But less than a year into his administration, faced with skyrocketing medical costs and the evident failure of both existing federal programs and Blue Cross to provide for the nation's health needs, he turned about and assigned a blue ribbon panel the job of studying national health insurance plans. The head of the panel is Walter McNerney, president of the National Blue Cross Association.

One reason for the sudden Presidential interest in health insurance is the increasingly evident failure of Medicaid (see chapter XI). But Blue Cross, the Medicaid of the middle-class, has been just as great a failure. The reasons lie in how the organization perceives its dual relationship with the public on the one hand, and with the providers of care on the other. The record shows that Blue Cross has turned into a major obstacle to decent health care for the American people.

Blue Cross was once a great social reform. For millions of Americans, faced with economic catastrophe if they got sick, it has meant that their hospital bills will in large part be paid. But Blue Cross has grown up into a monster. It is pricing itself out of people's reach, first with old people, whom it happily relinquished to Medicare in 1965, and now with lower-income people. By its abdication of responsibility for controlling medical costs, it is allowing everybody but the wealthy to be priced out of the medical care market. By its consistent submission to the hospitals, it has underwritten the survival of a hopelessly antiquated and unbalanced medical system. Even on its own turf—hospitalization insurance—Blue Cross is providing less and less for its subscribers, at an ever greater cost, while insisting that there are no alternatives. Finally, Blue Cross has distorted medical practice. For one example, it finances essentially only inpatient benefits; thus, ambulatory care, preventive medicine, and extended home care have received short shrift. For another, Blue Cross has great influence in the planning of medical care facilities. In the New York region, this influence has led to an acute shortage of hospital beds (see Chapter XIV).

These charges apply to all of the Blue Cross plans, to a greater or lesser extent, and are illustrated by the New York plan, called Associated Hospital Service (A.H.S.) With about eight million subscribers, A.H.S. is the largest Blue Cross plan in the nation. In May, 1969, A.H.S. asked the State Commissioner of Insurance to grant it permission to raise rates and make various changes in its way of operating. After vigorous public protest, all of the proposals except the rise in rates were turned down. A rate increase averaging forty-three percent (Blue Cross had asked fifty percent) was granted. However, what New York Blue Cross originally asked provides a good guide to the thinking of the men who control hospital financing. It also is a guide to the future, for what Blue Cross is denied this year it is likely to get the next time around.

In its request to the State, New York Blue Cross has essentially sought to abandon community rating and shift to experience rating. What this means can best be explained by example.

Suppose there are two groups of Blue Cross subscribers in a community. One group is made up of 900 generally young, white-collar workers in a bank. The second group is made up of 100 older, poorer machine operators in a garment factory. The members of the first group use relatively little hospitalization—an average of $100 worth of hospital services a year. The second group uses twice as much—$200 worth of hospital services a year, on the average. Under community rating, Blue Cross would charge the members of both groups the same rate for hospital insurance, even though the risk associated with individuals

in the two groups would differ. The rate would be calculated on the basis of the hospitalization experience of the
entire community. In the example, the 1,000 people in the
community use a total of $110,000 a year in hospital services
(900 people at $100 a year plus 100 people at $200 a year)
or an average of $110 per person per year. This amount, $110
(plus administrative expenses, of course), is what Blue
Cross would charge each person in the community for
insurance against hospitalization. The hospital expenses of
the entire membership are thus shared equally by the high-
risk groups and the low-risk groups. It was this policy of
charging a community rate, more than anything else,
which won for Blue Cross its reputation as a community
service rather than just another insurance company.

In recent years, however, Blue Cross has started acting
more like such private, profit-making insurance companies
as Aetna and Metropolitan. J. Douglas Colman, president
of Associated Hospital Service of New York, told the State
Insurance Department hearing on the 1969 rate hike proposal: "Small groups [that is, the better risks] must be
protected from being forced to subsidize large, self-
selected groups [that is, the poorer risks]." The *social* aspect of Blue Cross is thus forgotten. A.H.S. now offers
groups of more than a hundred members the option of
being experience-rated. In the example above, the employees of the bank would be charged $100 a year, and the
employees of the garment factory $200 a year. Low-risk
groups obviously benefit from an experience-rating, since
the rate charged them would not reflect the high hospital
utilization of poor-risk groups. The groups which remain
in the community-rated category are thus increasignly
those which need a lot of hospital care.

New York Blue Cross requested permission to divide

the remaining community-rated subscribers (currently about sixty percent of the total Blue Cross enrollment) into three major categories: direct-pay subscribers, subscribers in groups of over one hundred members, and subscribers in groups of under one hundred members. Each of these pools of subscribers would then be experience-rated. Worst hit by this method of setting rates would have been the direct-pay subscribers. This category contains many disabled, retired, unemployed, and self-employed workers, plus workers in small, marginal establishments. Some of these people have never qualified for a Blue Cross group policy. Others were covered by a group policy in a former place of employment, but upon leaving their jobs received a notice from Blue Cross saying: "The privilege of continuing your protection regardless of your employment status . . . is one of the many liberal features of your contract." Blue Cross requested a thirty-six to fifty-seven percent rate increase for this group. At the same time, it proposed to eliminate the most adequate contract available and force subscribers to replace it with a contract providing much less adequate coverage. The New York State Insurance Department refused to permit the contract change but did allow a thirty to sixty-five percent rate hike.

The members of the larger community-rated groups would also have been hurt by the Blue Cross proposal. Experience-rating has been available to these groups for some time now, and the groups which have chosen to remain in the community-rated category are generally the high-risk groups. Blue Cross proposed raising the rates as much as eighty-four percent for this group. By subdividing the community-rated groups into several experience-rated pools, based on size, Blue Cross was concentrating its rate increases on those most in need of services and least able to pay for them. The State denied permission to separately rate large and small groups, and granted rate increases of thirty-five to sixty-three percent for the various contracts. President Colman of A.H.S. was asked at a recent state legislative committee hearing what would happen to the people who could not afford the higher rates. He replied that they could fall back on Medicaid. Then he paused, reflecting on the series of cutbacks that have emasculated New York's Medicaid program and conceded that they couldn't rely on that, either. In fact, the only alternative for these people was to go to the municipal hospitals—and then welsh on their bills.

The attempted shift by Blue Cross to experience-rating is not confined to New York. In fact, few Blue Cross plans still retain as large a fraction of their subscribers on community rates as does the New York plan; many have no community-rated contracts at all. All of the plans are moving in this direction, if they're not already there. For example, the Connecticut Blue Cross Plan has recently filed for permission to institute a system of merit rating, i.e., experience-rating. Connecticut Blue Cross gives you a demerit if you get sick!

Meanwhile, Blue Cross benefits are deteriorating all over the country for all groups. For example, professional services, such as those of the anesthesiologist, the radiologist, and the pathologist used to be included as part of the hospital bill and thus were covered by Blue Cross. But, in recent years, these services have increasingly been billed separately, and, as a result, they fall under the less comprehensive coverage offered by Blue Shield. Thus, without any change in the language of the Blue Cross contract and without state regulatory action, subscribers are getting less and paying more. There also remain glaring deficiencies in the benefits offered by present contracts. For example, maternity care is essentially not covered (and is not covered at all for unmarried women), although this is the most common reason for hospitalization among young women.

Individual plans are in some cases making more direct cuts in benefits. In New York, for instance, Blue Cross wanted to follow the example of other plans by making certain subscribers pay part of the cost of their benefits themselves. This is called "coinsurance" or "copay" when the subscriber pays the first so many dollars of his bill. Both mechanisms represent an attempt by Blue Cross to shift some of the risk of medical costs to the subscriber.

Blue Cross' defense against its critics—that it is the helpless victim of rising hospital costs—holds water only if it is true that Blue Cross is powerless and that the increase in hospital costs is inevitable. But Blue Cross potentially has tremendous power to force hospitals to operate efficiently and rationally. In 1967, it paid directly about thirty-six percent of the bills for patient care in voluntary hospitals in southern New York State. In its role as the intermediary for Medicare, an additional thirty-two percent of the hospitals' total reimbursement passed through Blue Cross' hands. Thus Blue Cross, directly and indirectly, pays more than two-thirds of the hospitals' costs but makes virtually no attempt to control them.

For starters, Blue Cross pays the hospitals on a cost-plus basis. The hospitals say what they need to cover their costs, and Blue Cross pays up. Of course, Blue Cross claims that it scrutinizes hospital bills carefully and will only reimburse the hospitals for "reasonable" costs. This, it claims, has been significant in keeping costs down. Blue Cross, however, has a peculiar understanding of "reasonable:"

(1) Widely varying costs for providing very similar ser-

vices indicate that some hospitals are much more efficient than others. But to Blue Cross, regardless of the hospital's efficiency, incurred costs are "reasonable"—Blue Cross pays the bill.

(2) Blue Cross reimbursements to hospitals cover the cost of hiring labor relations lawyers and consultants to help keep hospital employees from organizing themselves into unions.

(3) Blue Cross reimbursements to hospitals cover the costs of expensive, but prestigious programs and equipment, even if unnecessary and underutilized.

Blue Cross' benefit structure has also helped promote overly high medical care costs for consumers. Benefits apply essentially only to inpatient hospital care. They do not cover use of outpatient departments or doctors' offices, nursing homes, chronic care homes, organized home care, etc., and so patients have a "disincentive" to use these types of care. It has been estimated that as many as twenty percent of the patients now in general hospitals could be treated just as well in these other ways, at great financial savings to the patient.

It is clear that really substantial savings in the cost of medical care depend on thorough-going rationalizations of the planning, running, and financing of hospitals (see chapter IX) and, indeed, of the entire medical care system. This, however, represents a fundamental challenge to the power of the men who presently plan and run the hospitals. And this is exactly what Blue Cross has shown itself unwilling to do.

Blue Cross has undertaken energetic action to control costs in one way. In the last decade, prodded by federal legislation, regional planning agencies for health facilities have sprung up throughout the country (see chapter XIV).

These agencies are supposed to scrutinize all plans for new hospital construction, as well as plans for modernization or expansion of existing facilities, in order to prevent unnecessary duplication. In some places the planning agencies' decisions are binding, in others, only advisory. Blue Cross is a great proponent of this planning movement. As of late 1968, thirty of the seventy-five Blue Cross plans were actively supporting local health planning councils, and the national Blue Cross Association was considering making such participation mandatory for all plans. The New York Blue Cross gives $100,000 a year to the Health and Hospital Planning Council of Southern New York (H.H.P.C. the agency which, according to state law, must approve all projected hospital construction in the area), making Blue Cross H.H.P.C.'s largest nongovernmental contributor. And no less than eight Blue Cross trustees and officers sit on the H.H.P.C. Board of Trustees (five of them are H.H.P.C. officers as well).

What's in it for Blue Cross? Well, you can't use more hospital beds than exist, so the absolute upper limit on Blue Cross' liability is set by the number of hospital beds available to its subscribers. Hence, through its participation in planning councils, Blue Cross seeks to limit the number of hospital beds in the area. This is the way Blue Cross described its position on health planning in New York when it filed for its 1969 rate increase with the New York State Insurance Commissioner:

> There is clear evidence that the amount of hospital care, and, therefore, the community's total hospital bill, including that of A.H.S. [New York Blue Cross] subscribers, is materially influenced by the amount of hospital facilities available for use. Hospital utilization among A.H.S. subscribers was appreciably lower than for those in other Blue Cross plans. . . . This

lower utilization reflects the active support A.H.S. has given the concept of area-wide planning for hospital facilities. . . . A.H.S.'s active participation in these activities . . . has indeed "paid off" both for its subscribers and for the community at large.

In other words, Blue Cross has done its best to make hospital beds hard to find. In 1969, average occupancy rates in voluntary hospitals in New York City soared into the ninety percent-and-up range, the highest in the country, and it became difficult to get a hospital bed even in emergencies. One city doctor claims ironically that he's going to cancel his Blue Cross coverage. If you have a heart attack, he points out, the first twenty-four hours are crucial. And if hospitals are so crowded that you can't get in immediately, he reasons, you may be just as well off recuperating at home—if you live. This is what Blue Cross means by a cost-control measure that has "paid off."

Blue Cross fails to control hospital costs for its subscribers simply because Blue Cross is controlled by the hospital establishment. The hospitals created it during the Depression to ensure that their bills would be paid. The trademark Blue Cross itself is owned by the American Hospital Association. The influence of the hospitals in Blue Cross can be seen in the way the plans are controlled. Subscribers are not stockholders in Blue Cross: neither law nor custom gives them any say whatsoever in how Blue Cross is managed. The typical plan provides for a self-recruited board of trustees on which the medical industry holds a majority of seats. In no case do the subscribers have a vote in choosing the trustees. The common pattern is for doctors to hold one third of the seats, hospital administrators and trustees another third, and lay representatives the other third. In some plans, the local medical society and the hospital association choose their trustees, and those trustees, in turn, choose the public representatives. In southern New York, all Blue Cross directors are elected by a corporation. As of January 1970, of the thirty-four voting members of the corporation, no less than twenty are hospital officials and trustees, officials of the hospital-dominated Health and Hospital Planning Council, physicians, or officials of the voluntary hospitals' fund-raising front, the United Hospital Fund. More than half of the remaining members are big businessmen. Thus, the public representatives on the Blue Cross board are not only usually in the minority, but they are chosen by the hospital-medical establishment. Under these circumstances, it is rare to hear a critical voice on the board.

New York has fourteen consumer representatives on its twenty-five-member board, but few of them look even remotely like spokesmen for the subscribers. Eight members are big businessmen (including representatives from Con Edison, International Nickel, A.T. & T., a Wall Street law firm, and a Wall Street broker). Five are labor leaders, but at least two of these are from unions which have few members covered by Blue Cross. There are several educators, judges, and City officials who do not represent anyone except themselves. Ten board members come from the hospital-medical establishment (including two of the businessmen, who sit on hospital boards, and the vice-president and Dean of the School of Medicine at Mount Sinai Medical Center, who is listed by Blue Cross as representing the "general public").

The result is, in New York and elsewhere, that when hospitals negotiate their reimbursement contracts with Blue Cross, they are essentially negotiating with themselves. Belief that cost-cutting pressure on the hospitals will result from such negotiations is much like believing, along with the A.M.A., that doctors can regulate physicians' fees in the public interest. As the representative of the International Union of Electrical Workers said at the hearings on the 1969 New York Blue Cross rate increase: "Why hasn't A.H.S. [Blue Cross] been the voice of the consumer? The reason is that A.H.S. is dominated by people with an interest in medical income."

Another source of the hospital's control over Blue Cross is their contracts with the insurance organization. Blue Cross does not pay the hospital's bill to the individual patient. Rather, it has a contract with the hospital specifying that Blue Cross will pay the hospital a certain allowable cost for each day of hospital service used by a Blue Cross subscriber. The allowable cost which Blue Cross will pay is less than the total cost of the hospital of providing service. Such items as research overhead, educational costs for a residency or intern program, or for a hospital school of nursing, and the cost of providing service for patients who fail to pay their bills are not included in Blue Cross payments, although part of those costs would be included in the bill of a person paying his hospital bill himself or with the aid of a commercial insurance policy. The advantage to the hospitals of giving Blue Cross this special rate is that they are assured, through Blue Cross, a stable income from the many patients who might otherwise fail to pay their bills. But it also means that the hospitals have an effective club over Blue Cross: they can withdraw the preferential rate they offer to Blue Cross and demand that Blue Cross pay them their full charges. Blue Cross guarantees its subscribers payment for X days of hospitalization. So if any substantial number of hospitals in a given area took this course, Blue Cross would either have to pay the hospitals their full charges or else default on paying full benefits for patients in these hospitals. Either course would destroy Blue Cross' competitive position with respect to the commercial health insurance companies.

In at least one instance, hospitals have made successful use of this weapon. In Philadelphia in the late 1950s, Blue Cross got uppity and put the long-range interest of its subscribers (and of its own finances) ahead of the immediate interests of the hospitals. It tried to impose a reimbursement formula on the hospitals which would force them to operate more efficiently. In 1959 about half of the hospitals in the area refused to renew their contracts with Blue Cross. After prolonged negotiations, Blue Cross knuckled under and abandoned the cost-controlling payment scheme for a plan based on "full and equitable" costs of each institution.

A petty example illustrates Blue Cross' close relationship with the hospitals. The day after New York Blue Cross filed its rate increase proposal with the State Department of Insurance, a letter went out from Blue Cross Vice President Mark A. Freedman to administrators of its member hospitals. He enclosed a copy of the filing and a lengthy question-and-answer sheet explaining it. But three months later, Blue Cross had still not seen fit to notify its subscribers that a rate increase was in the works.

The alliance of Blue Cross and the hospitals was also evident at the hearings held by the New York State Insurance Superintendent on August 4, 1969. In opposition to the Blue Cross proposal was every group that could be construed as representing consumers: unions, such as the International Union of Electrical Workers, Teamsters Joint Council 16, the Drug and Hospital Workers, and the Sanitationmen's Union; voluntary community service groups; and the New York City Department of Consumer Affairs and Department of Health. Speaking in support of Blue Cross were only the hospital administrators and Blue Cross itself.

If Blue Cross fails to represent the public with respect to the hospitals, the public agencies which regulate Blue Cross don't help much either. Closeness between Blue Cross and the public officials who supposedly regulate it, encouraged by the possibility of a prestigious Blue Cross position as a reward later on, is said to be quite common. For example, lawyer Thomas Thacher was New York State Superintendent of Insurance from 1959 to 1963. Blue Cross critics allege that during his term in the Insurance Department, Thacher was extraordinarily sympathetic to some of Blue Cross' legally more questionable demands and practices. Thacher now sits on the board of New York Blue Cross.

Another example is a Pennsylvania Insurance Commissioner and his daughter who were given posts with the Blue Cross Association in the mid-1950s. Important insurance commissioners are also often invited to the annual Blue Cross Association meetings, there to be wined and dined in return for a brief speech. And when the 1969 New York Blue Cross rate hike was subsequently challeged in court, a State Supreme Court justice summed up relations between Blue Cross and the Department of Insurance by scolding State Insurance Commissioner Richard Stewart for his "arbitrary, capricious, hasty, and ill-advised" approval of the rate increase. Stewart had, to be sure, turned down many of Blue Cross' proposals and trimmed its rate proposal. But observers of past Blue Cross rate increase requests saw a familiar pattern. The hearings, they say, were merely group therapy for the opposition. Blue Cross asks for an outrageous amount, the charade of the hearing is played out, and the insurance commissioner grants a smaller, but still stupendous, increase. Blue Cross gets what it expected and the public is led to think that the regulatory agencies are really looking out for consumer interests after all.

Periodic gusts of public dissatisfaction have not slowed the impressive growth of Blue Cross. Like other nonprofit institutions, such as universities and medical schools, Blue Cross is forever seeking to expand its operations. It behaves like a hungry corporation, the difference being that its profits are all plowed back into the business. Blue Cross has its sights set on controlling any future expansion of Medicaid or a national health insurance plan, both of which become more probable as the health crisis worsens. The prospects for Blue Cross are rosy. President Nixon's appointment of Walter McNerney, president of the Blue Cross Association, as head of the "Task Force on Medicaid and Related Programs" was read by many as auguring a proposal featuring Blue Cross management of Medicaid.

The task force was also charged with making proposals for a national health insurance system. According to Health, Education and Welfare officials, the plan that is likely to emerge would use federal money along with pay-roll taxes on employers and employees to buy insurance from private companies. Blue Cross, with its favored position in the hospitals, would have the inside track and a good prospect of monopolizing the business.

XI

MEDICAID:

KILLERS OF THE DREAM

Medicaid began in 1966 just as the war in Vietnam hit full stride. Medicaid began to die two years ($100 billion of war effort) later. For those few months in between, for a couple of million New Yorkers, health care was free. Health care —if you could find it—was a right. Teeth were filled, glasses were fitted, hearts were checked in a long, long overdue medical shopping spree.

Medicaid, Title 19 of the 1965 Social Security Amendments, was the sleeper amendment adopted by Congress along with Medicare, Title 18. It was to be a program of federal matching grants to states that chose to provide medical services to certain categories of welfare recipients —the blind, the disabled, the aged, and parents of dependent children. The soaring costs of the program, however, especially in the few states like New York which set high income eligibility limits, made Congress see red. In 1967, Congress amended the law to make it crystal clear that it had not intended Medicaid to be anything more than welfare medicine. The amendments placed a ceiling on the family incomes above which federal matching funds would not be available. States would no longer receive reimbursement for those people whose incomes were greater than 133 percent of the standard state welfare grant.

With such half-hearted Federal participation, the program was doomed. Though Medicaid had originally seemed to promise that everyone who needed medical care would be able to pay for it, the states were not eager to create the necessary programs while Congress was unwilling to kick in the money. Meanwhile, the costs of even the truncated programs that remained were soaring, and state after state was forced to tighten up on eligibility requirements. One state, New Mexico, at one point decided to drop out of the program entirely.

It's all, or almost all, over now, and time to take a cold, hard look at Medicaid. What did it buy? How much did it cost? Would we do it again if we had the money? New York, which had a heavier commitment to health care for the poor to begin with, and which embraced Medicaid like a long lost brother, fell the hardest. By the depth of its fall, it reveals most clearly what happened in other cities as well.

The answers echoing from the frontlines are bitter. "Medicaid set health care in New York City back thirty years," says one veteran hospital physician. "Now, we're just picking up the pieces." Starting in late 1966, Medicaid hit New York City's medical marketplace like a flash flood. What's left is an altogether new game.

(1) The stakes are higher. Uncontrolled medical inflation shoved millions of New Yorkers into medical indigency and onto the brink of welfare.

(2) The rules are different. The city government's historic role was the provision of care for both the indigent and the medically indigent—those too rich for welfare and too poor for health care. Now the city's commitment extends not a penny past the state capitol's nineteenth cen-

tury definitions of poverty. What's more, the city's ability
to guarantee care, as opposed to just money for care, has
deteriorated. Municipal hospital budgets have been starved
to feed the rising cost of care in the private hospitals.

(3) There are fewer players. Squeezed beteeen the rising
costs of care and sinking definitions of medical indigency,
thousands of consumers have simply vanished from the
medical care scene.

There were no good old days in the city's health history,
but the old days were not that bad, either. Before Medicaid, New York City's commitment to health care for the
poor was heavier than that of any other city in the country.
The city operated twenty-one municipal hospitals, all of
which offered inpatient and clinic care free to the medically indigent, and over thirty health centers, which offered free preventive care to everyone.

Because of these comparatively high existing standards,
New York City was the pace setter (and eventually the
bank buster) for Medicaid nationally. New York State set
its income eligibility limit at $6000 a year for a family of
four, compared to the runner-up, California, with $3900.
For the eligible, there was a full range of services, twice as
many as mandated by federal law. Rich as this program
later seemed to many conservative congressmen, it was
not quantitatively much different from what New York
City had offered before.

Medicaid was different, though, in two important ways.
For the poor, Medicaid meant not just guaranteed health
care but a free choice of the source of care. Patients would
be free to "spend" their benefits at either city or private
facilities. For the city, Medicaid meant an initially unlimited amount of state and federal matching money for
health expenses. Except for A.M.A.-oriented profession-

als, everyone agreed that these two features of Medicaid guaranteed an end to charity care, and the beginning of an age in which everyone would enjoy the mainstream of modern medicine. Everyone did not agree, however, on how this would all come about. Many private medical leaders saw the change occurring as people exercised their free choice, thinking they would obviously opt for private, rather than city facilities. Gradually the city hospitals would empty out, and the city would have no choice but to turn the buildings over to the private sector.

Officials in Mayor Lindsay's newly formed Health Services Administration (H.S.A.)* sized up the situation somewhat differently. H.S.A.'s 1966-67 chief, Dr. Howard Brown, focused on the financial aspect of Medicaid. He saw that the new state and federal money could be used to upgrade municipal facilities, by renovating city hospitals and creating a host of new "Neighborhood Family Care Centers" along the lines of the federal antipoverty program's comprehensive health care centers. At the same time, the immense new quantities of money could be used as a lever on the private sector—to raise the standards of private hospital and physician care, and to insure that all doors would be open to the sick poor.

For all these good intentions, Medicaid hit the city government almost wholly unprepared. In spite of the enormous weight of the administrative machinery brought to bear on Medicaid, no one sat on top, watching where the money was going and who was getting what for it. The

---

*H.S.A. is a "super-agency" set up in 1966 to integrate the city's previously separate health agencies: the Departments of Health and Hospitals, the Community Mental Health Board, and the Office of the Chief Medical Examiner.

city agency which stood to gain (or lose) the most with Medicaid, the Department of Hospitals, took a wait-and-see attitude. It made no attempts to capture Medicaid money for its own underfinanced facilities—through insuring efficient enrollment of patients, and by offering more personalized service in order to attract Medicaid eligibles. Perhaps the Department of Hospitals was waiting to see if all the city patients would eventually drift off to the private sector.

Most of the people never made it to the private sector. Utilization of the municipal hospitals has declined since Medicaid began, but far less than was initially expected. Today the city hospitals are still overcrowded in relation to the size of their staffs, and are still the major provider of medical care for the poor.

The interesting question is not "how many people did the city hospitals lose?" but "what did people who left them gain?" Where did they go and what services did they find there? The only hard data we have are the changes in municipal hospital utilization. The story they tell about Medicaid is not an altogether happy one.

The decline in inpatient utilization. People began deserting city beds when the Medicare program began, and continued when Medicaid started. At the same time, voluntary and proprietary hospitals reported gains in utilization. The exodus from the city to the private sector stopped, though, in October 1967, when the city had so far experienced only a four percent decline in patient-days. At this point the private hospitals apparently achieved near-maximum occupancy rates, and stopped crowding in Medicaid and Medicare patients. Comparing 1966 and 1967, voluntary occupancy rates rose from eighty-four to eighty-six percent, proprietary rates rose from seventy-nine to eighty-five percent, and municipal rates fell from seventy-seven to seventy-five percent.

This pattern of occupancy rates has been economically unhealthy for the city hospital system. Empty beds are almost as expensive to maintain as full beds, and of course, empty beds don't bring in any Medicaid or Medicare money. Still, hospitals have to leave some beds empty in case of emergencies. In effect, the municipal hospital system now serves as the safety margin for the entire private sector; some voluntary hospitals have let their occupancy rates soar over ninety percent, knowing that the municipal hospitals can absorb any occasional overflows.

The decline in municipal OPD (Outpatient Department) utilization. It was in outpatient services that the greatest decline in utilization was expected, since over ninety percent of the OPD visitors were Medicaid-eligible in 1967, hence free to find their own family physicians. Some planners in H.S.A. optimistically expected that Medicaid would decompress the municipal OPDs to such a point that extensive renovation and reorganization could be undertaken. But the decline in OPD utilization was disappointing. First, it was far smaller than expected. Second, at least part of the drop in municipal OPD use cannot be attributed to a shift to voluntary hospital OPDs, private doctors, or any health facilities.

The second point emerged only recently, when the Department of Hospitals released a careful, month-by-month statistical analysis of OPD utilization. They found that OPD use stopped rising, for the first time in about six years, in early 1967, when Medicaid enrollment began to get underway. The early '67 decrease was not statistically significant (given the wide seasonal fluctuations in OPD use) until July 1967. This was the month when, for the first time in New York City history, fees were charged in municipal OPDs.

The purpose of the 1967 eight-dollar clinic fee was to encourage people to enroll in Medicaid. Instead it seems to have discouraged a great many people from using the municipal clinics. Whether the people who left the municipal clinics were Medicaid-ineligibles who couldn't afford the fee, or Medicaid-eligibles who had not yet enrolled and were frightened by the fees, is impossible to say. Hospital statisticians point out that most of the OPD visits lost by the city hospitals did not show up as increased visits to voluntary hospitals. They and many clinic doctors fear that these people were simply driven out of the medical marketplace.

One thing is clear: people did not rush out of the municipal OPD's to exercise their right to a free choice of medical care. They left rather sluggishly, prodded by the eight-dollar, then eleven-dollar fees. Ignorance and apathy, the stock explanations of the health habits of the poor, cannot take the blame. Most people would have preferred something better than clinic care. For instance, a 1965 survey of municipal OPD users found that, if money were not a problem, thirty-eight percent of the patients would have preferred a private doctor, and seventeen percent would have preferred some other hospital. Thus, almost sixty percent of the OPD users might have been expected to leave in 1967. However, the same survey showed that only eighteen percent of the OPD users had recently used a private doctor. Another thirty-three percent had no source of care except the city hospital OPD they were interviewed in. This is not surprising. For many people, despite Medicaid, no alternatives were available. Even though New York has more doctors per capita than any other city in the nation. some of its ghetto areas have fewer than ten practicing general practitioners per 100,000 people—a doctor density rivaling that of rural Mississippi. Furthermore, sixty percent of the New York City general practitioners chose to turn Medicaid patients away from their offices.

Who benefited from the so-called free choice offered by Medicaid? No doubt thousands of people were able to use a doctor's office in their neighborhood, rather than a distant municipal OPD. But for many more people, the only free choice was whether to get care in the municipal OPD or not to get care at all. Park Avenue aside, New York simply doesn't have a wealth of ambulatory care resources to choose from.

Medicaid, even at its height, then, failed to free the poor from the reign of poorhouse medicine. Then, in 1967, in response to the unexpectedly high costs, Congress placed a ceiling on the federal responsibility under the Medicaid program. As federal support faded, New York State also cut back on its commitment. In March 1968 the legislature cut the upper income eligibility limits from $6000 for a family of four to $5300, and excluded from the program almost all people between the ages of twenty-one and sixty-four other than welfare recipients, the disabled, and the blind. Together with a second set of cuts in 1969, more than 1.2 million New York City residents were kicked off the Medicaid rolls.

Despite the fears of liberals, no one rioted. It was not that the poor were uninterested in medical care. They were just not impressed by Medicaid. In many respects, it was the private providers, far more than the consumers, who benefited from Medicaid's funds, and it was the providers who raised the loudest protest at the cutback. In fact, the Health and Hospital Planning Council, the mouthpiece of the city's private medical establishment, was so moved by the 1968 cutback that it actually called (from its posh east side offices) for public demonstrations.

The real tragedy of the March 1968 cutbacks was not immediately apparent. That spring and early summer, the city braced itself for a massive influx of patients returning to the Municipal hospitals. Months passed, and hospital utilization rates continued to drop. Downtown at the city Department of Hospitals, health planners were baffled. The visit load at municipal OPDs was dropping more rapidly than ever before. Both inpatient and outpatient loads at private hospitals were dropping too, so no new shift was underway.

The mystery of the disappearing patients was finally cleared up by interns and residents at Bronx Municipal Hospital's pediatric clinic. The ex-Medicaid patients were not coming to the municipal clinics because they couldn't afford the fee, which had by this time soared to sixteen dollars. In an unprecendented patients' rights protest, hospital house staff publicly told their patients not to pay, and to mail the bills to Hospitals Commissioner Terenzio. In response to the protest, clinic fees were reset on a scale which slides from two dollars to sixteen dollars. Even with these supposedly nominal fees, many clinic doctors are alarmed at continuing declines in clinic utilization. People are saving by skipping vital preventive services such as prenatal check-ups.

Even though Medicaid failed to move charity patients into the mainstream of private medical practice, we might still expect that the newly available funds would have helped refurbish the city's decaying public hospital system. Medicaid brought hundreds of millions of state and federal health dollars into New York City. Where has all the money gone? Some rough impressions, pieced together from the city budget and Health Department figures are:

About eighty percent goes to hospitals of all kinds. Less than seven percent goes to family doctors. The rest is for dentists, drugs, X-rays, and miscellaneous items.

Less than a third (somewhat over $200 million) goes to the city hospitals (although they cost about $400 million per year to run and almost all their patients are Medicaid eligible).

About half goes to private hospitals and nursing homes.

Altogether about a third goes for items and services which are sold at a profit: drugs, nursing home, and proprietary hospital care.

The peculiar thing about Medicaid money is that the more you spend, the less it's worth. In the first year of the Medicaid (and Medicare) program, doctors' fees rose 2.4 times as fast as the overall cost of living. Hospital costs rose four times as fast as the cost of living. A reasonable increase in hospital prices should have been expected in the late '60s —because of higher wages for nonprofessionals, the high costs of new life-saving equipment, etc. But costs never would have risen so high so fast without Medicaid and Medicare. According to law, Medicaid must pay each hospital exactly what that hospital claims as its cost for rendering a service.

The trouble with this is that it is uncontrollably expensive. As a former administrator of the city's Medicaid program pointed out, under Medicaid, there's no incentive for a hospital to be efficient. It was because of the wildly and irresponsibly escalating hospital costs—not because of abuse by patients or fee-hustling by private doctors—that Congress slashed Medicaid in 1968.

Initially, Medicaid was seen as easing the city's load in an already heavy commitment to health spending. But under the Medicaid program, the city was required to match state and federal funds. Because of unexpectedly high costs, Medicaid turned out to be a major new drain on the city tax dollar. The city found itself committed to paying thirty percent of the bill, which rose higher every month. Most of the money did not return to city facilities; it flowed out to the private sector through an open-ended account. As the Mayor pointed out in his 1969 budget message, seventy-one percent of all the state and federal funds brought into the city by Medicaid since 1966 went to the private sector. Only twenty-nine percent went to city hospitals.

The city hospitals not only failed to profit from Medicaid, they have probably suffered a net loss. Under Medicaid, the city could do little—that is, little which would not have involved stepping on politically sensitive toes—to check the flow of funds to the private sector. The only politically safe way of controlling the costs of the Medicaid program was to clamp down on funds for the municipal hospitals. This was done, in part, by diverting Medicaid funds which were due to the city hospitals to other city departments. State Senator Seymour Thaler estimates that the city Budget Bureau has been "saving" about 100 million Medicaid dollars earned by city hospitals annually by plowing them into the city's treasury.

What is happening then, is a far-reaching change in the city's entire pattern of health spending. In 1966, less than twenty-five percent of the city's health budget was allotted to private providers. Now the figure is up to forty percent, and if amounts paid to voluntary hospitals to staff city hospitals were included, one would find that over half the city health dollar goes to the private sector. The problem is not that this money is handed over to the private sector, but that it is handed over with virtually no strings attached. The great bulk of the money flows to private institutions for services which are not monitored, evaluated, or measured by any public agency. Increasingly, the city plays the passive role of a conduit for health funds; guaranteeing payment to the private providers, but guaranteeing nothing to the consumers.

The promise of Medicaid was a new era of health care in New York City. The new state and federal funds could have been used as a lever to force a reorientation of private institutional medicine in the public interest: the abolition of wards, the reorganization of clinics to ensure continuity of care, and a new emphasis on preventive and ambulatory care. Medicaid money could also have been used directly, to upgrade municipal hospitals and to finance scores of neighborhood health centers.

The reality of Medicaid was that services which had once been free now carried a price tag. Almost all of the twenty or so neighborhood health centers which the city had promised to build with Medicaid funds failed to grow out of the preplanning stage. For most Medicaid recipients, Medicaid brought no new services (with the exception of dentistry in some neighborhoods) and no higher quality in the old. Meanwhile, for the Medicaid money recipients, private hospitals, and nursing homes, Medicaid was a windfall.

The residue of Medicaid, now that it has been cut to a near-meaningless level, is the wreckage of the city's forty-year-old public health and hospital system. The city has less to offer, to fewer people and at greater cost, than at any other time since the Depression.

XII

NATIONAL HEALTH INSURANCE:

THE GREAT LEAP SIDEWAYS

What Otto von Bismarck did for Germany in the 1880s, Richard Nixon is trying to do for the United States in the 1970s. Faced with rising social unrest, the Iron Chancellor looked for solutions to various social problems through a series of welfare laws. One of them became the world's first national health insurance system. Almost ninety years later, Nixon, too, faces the necessity of "solving" the social crises which are nurturing the new student, community, and worker insurgencies. One of the crises he sees is in the delivery of health care. And, like his Teutonic predecessor, the President, along with powerful business, labor, and health establishment forces may turn toward national health insurance.

In fact, however, there are not one but two health crises. The crisis felt by the users of medical services is the failure of the present system to deliver adequate health care at any price. Black and Puerto Rican community groups are demanding community control over health institutions which they perceive to be wholly unaccountable to the people they serve and wholly unresponsive to the pressing health needs of the community. Medical care, they say, is fragmented, and is isolated from the social, economic, and environmental sources of pathology. Furthermore, they maintain that patients are experimented on and used as teaching material. The doctors' priorities come first, and the patients' needs run a poor second.

Increasingly the middle class is beginning to raise many of the same questions, led on by soaring costs, long waits in overcrowded doctors' waiting rooms, and the growing awareness that despite the wonders of heart transplants, it is increasingly difficult to find a doctor to treat anything as mundane as arthritis or asthma.

Those who provide and pay for health care face a different crisis—the breakdown of the old systems of financing. The hospitals find themselves near collapse as costs skyrocket and financing fails to keep up. This threatens not only the institutions themselves, but also the multi-billion-dollar drug and hospital supply companies who depend on the hospitals as a retail outlet for their products. At the same time that the hospitals weep because of inadequate funds, the providers of funds groan under the weight of the hospitals. Blue Cross is forced to raise its rates and face its enraged subscribers. The trade unions find themselves allocating an ever-increasing portion of wage hikes merely to maintain their present level of health benefits. Employee health plans cut an ever bigger bite out of corporate profits. Even the government feels the pinch as Medicare and Medicaid costs knock the budget for a loop.

Since the providers and financiers of medical care feel only part of the crisis—the part concerning the financing of medical care—it is little wonder that their solution to the crisis concerns only that. The various plans for health insurance proposed by such various groups and figures as the A.M.A., Walter Reuther, the A.F.L.-C.I.O., Nelson Rockefeller, Blue Cross President Walter McNerney, the

American Hospital Association, and Senators Jacob Javits and Edward Kennedy are all simply programs to put the financing of medical care on a sounder basis. The issues which are debated—coverage, benefits, sources of financing, administrative mechanisms, etc.—all attempt to answer the question of how to finance existing health services. None of the proposals seriously confront other parts of the crisis—the basic issues of the organization of delivery systems, the relationship between the providers and recipients of care, power in the health delivery system, or priorities in the system.

Proposals for national health insurance are nothing new in the nation's health history. In 1914, the American Association for Labor Legislation drafted a model plan and submitted it to state legislatures across the country; not a single state acted. In 1935, national health insurance was successfully kept out of the Social Security Act, largely by A.M.A. pressure. Another plan, the Wagner-Murray-Dingle Bill, was proposed in 1943 without administration support and never made it out of congressional committee. Again, in 1948, the bill was pushed, this time with backing from President Truman, only to die in committee. It was only in 1965, by limiting coverage to the elderly, that a nationwide health insurance scheme, Medicare, was adopted.

What is new about the current wave of national health insurance proposals is the strength of the army forming to force them through. On the one flank is the public, led on by the mass media to expect ever-greater miracles from the medical magicians, but increasingly frustrated in their ability to obtain even ordinary nostrums. On the other flank is labor, management, the hospitals, Blue Cross, the companies that manufacture and sell hospital supplies, and local and state governments, each faced with an increasingly serious set of problems growing out of the horse-and-buggy methods of financing medical services, each seeing one or another brand of national health insurance as a solution to its own special health care crisis.

Labor wants national health insurance to eliminate the hassle at the bargaining table over health fringe benefits, which have taken increasingly large bites out of the wage package. In 1965, for example, in the steel industry, nineteen cents an hour, or four percent of the average steel worker's total wages and benefits, went for health and life insurance. Today, because medical prices have gone up two to three times as fast as prices in general, as much as eight to ten percent of any new wage and benefit package would have to go to health and life insurance, just to maintain the existing health benefits. At a time when the real disposable income of American workers has stopped growing for a several-year period for the first time in twenty years (due largely to inflation and increased taxes because of the Vietnam war), labor is desperate to find ways to augment workers' wages. Relegating health insurance to the government leaves more dollars and cents for wage increases.

Management also wants national health insurance, because health insurance premiums have become a significant and rapidly rising component of their overall labor costs. Businesses would like to stabilize the contribution they make for their employees' health care: predictability of costs permits planning for larger profits. In addition, national health insurance may shift part of management's labor costs (i.e., the health insurance component) onto government, leading to greater profits. This shift of labor costs from management to government would be limited to those large industrial employers whom labor has already compelled to make substantial contributions to health insurance. The marginal, small shop or agricultural employer who now makes little or no contribution to health insurance for his employees, may find that national health insurance increases his labor costs. While management is not unified on the issue of national health insurance, those that count (big business and industry) seem more and more in favor of it.

Of the medical-industrial complex (see chapter VII), the hospital supply and equipment companies, the medical electronics and computer companies, and those at least drug companies which are diversified into hospital supplies, all would benefit from national health insurance. Their experience with Medicare and Medicaid has been profitable. As *Value Line Investment Survey* pointed out in mid-1967, because of programs like Medicare the hospital supply industry is "operating in a sector of the economy that is virtually recession-proof."

For the voluntary (private, nonprofit) hospitals almost any program of national health insurance would be better than the present Medicaid program. Eligibility has become so restricted under Medicaid that many patients are no longer covered. That leaves the hospitals stuck with the bills of patients who are too rich for Medicaid but too poor to pay (and too sick to turn away). A national health insurance program allows the possibility of universal coverage without eligibility restrictions. Equally important, national health insurance would stabilize hospital income by guaranteeing a certain level of reimbursement. Government will be reluctant to cut a program that affects a large cross-section of Americans. Of course, the voluntaries would prefer a national health insurance plan which merely subsidized their operations with minimal interference from government. But, for them, almost any form of national health insurance would be better than none.

Blue Cross/Blue Shield, the fiscal intermediary of the voluntary hospitals, wants a particular brand of national health insurance, one that would expand Blue Cross hegemony over the health insurance market. Although Blue Cross enrollment has flowered over the last decades, its percentage of the health insurance market has been declining. In 1945, Blue Cross insured sixty-one percent of the hospital insurance market compared to thirty-three percent by the commercial insurance companies. Today, that figure is reversed for the population under age sixty-five, with Blue Cross garnering only thirty-four percent of the hospital insurance market compared to sixty percent by the commercial insurance companies. However, Medicare and Medicaid represented a big boost to Blue Cross, since virtually every state turned over administration of their programs to Blue Cross. It is just such a relationship to national health insurance that Blue Cross wishes to develop. With Walter McNerney, President of the Blue Cross Association of America, as chairman of the presidential task force assigned to investigate national health insurance, there is little doubt that Blue Cross' interests will be represented.

Finally, local and state governments see rising costs for their health programs (state and city hospitals, Medicaid, etc.) as an unlimited drain on already scarce funds. Any program that shifts part of the burden off their backs is welcome. As a result, even the most ardent states' righters voted enthusiastically to support New York Governor Nelson Rockefeller's National Health Insurance proposals at the 1969 National Governors' Conference.

In sum, labor, management, parts of the medical-industrial complex, the voluntary hospitals, Blue Cross, and local governments all want some form of national health insurance. This newly forming coalition is based on the power and pecuniary needs of these groups rather than the health needs of the public. Such a coalition is coming into being for the first time only now, explaining in part the recurrent failures to enact national health insurance in America. The coalescence of these forces now spells not only the inevitability of national health insurance, but also suggests the shape and form it will take.

Three major types of plan have been proposed for universal or national health insurance. Each plan is best designated after the name of the individual or group that came out with it first: the A.M.A. Plan, the Rockefeller Plan, and the Reuther Plan.

The A.M.A. Plan is not really a program of national health insurance at all. Rather, it is a national system of incentives to encourage individuals to *voluntarily* purchase private (commercial or Blue Cross) health insurance. The incentive would be in the form of an income tax credit. (Hence the plan is called "medicredit" by the A.M.A.'s public relations men.) An individual who purchased health insurance would have the right to deduct a certain fraction of the insurance premiums from the income taxes he pays the federal government. The percentage would depend on how much tax he owed. Poor people (the thirty percent of the population with the lowest tax liability) would receive vouchers entitling them to purchase health insurance at government expense. People who are slightly better off might be able to count seventy percent of the dollars they pay for health insurance as if they were dollars paid in taxes. Still richer people would get credit for a smaller percentage of their premiums, while people with a very high income, and hence a very high tax liability, would get no tax credit at all. In effect, the government would be paying for a variable fraction of the health insurance premiums individuals chose to buy—directly for the very poor and indirectly, by foregoing part of its tax revenues, for everyone else.

The A.M.A. Plan would interfere least with the way medicine is practiced in the country. There would be no cost controls and no new administrative apparatus (both patients and providers would continue to deal directly with insurance companies). Commercial insurance companies are expected to favor the A.M.A. Plan or some variation of it, which subsidizes their customers while entailing little risk of regulation for them.

The Rockefeller Plan revolves around mandatory purchase of private health insurance (Blue Cross, H.I.P. or a commercial policy). It differs from the A.M.A. Plan primarily because it is compulsory (which entitles it to the label "universal health insurance"). Insurance premiums for working people would be paid by employer and employee contributions. The unemployed and the poor would have their premiums paid by the government out of general tax revenues. Medicare would continue as it is. As with the A.M.A. Plan, there would be little need for new administrative apparatus, since patients and providers would deal directly with private insurance companies. With Blue Cross and commercial insurance companies running the show, cost controls are likely to be minimal.

Although the American Hospital Association (A.H.A.) representing 7,000 voluntary hospitals and nursing homes, has not released their plan for national health insurance at this writing, it is almost certain that they will favor a Rockefeller-type plan. Ray Brown, past president of the A.H.A., has been quoted in a late 1969 issue of a hospital journal: "We've got to find the additional support for our hospital system, and I think, our whole medical care system, in the private sector. The one way to do this is to . . . set a national standard for minimum benefits for health coverage, then mandate . . . that every employer have this minimum coverage for everyone that he employs."

It is expected that the McNerney task force, representing Blue Cross, if it proposes anything beyond patching up Medicaid, will also support a Rockefeller-type plan. And the National Governors' Conference of 1969 has already come out in favor of the Rockefeller Plan.

The Reuther Plan for national (rather than universal) health insurance would be "an integral part of the national social insurance system." It would be compulsory health insurance for everyone, with the government acting as the insurer. The program would supplant most of the coverage now offered by private companies (Blue Cross and the commercials). The Reuther Plan would be paid for by employer, employee, and government contributions: tentatively, two-thirds of the cost would come from employer-employee contributions, while one-third would come from general tax revenues. Medicaid would be eliminated, and Medicare would be integrated into the national plan. The Reuther Plan, in contradistinction to the A.M.A. and Rockefeller plans, would require a new administrative apparatus resembling that for Medicare. Whether the government would administer the entire program itself or would turn over much of this role to private companies such as Blue Cross (as they do with Medicare) remains to be decided.

The Reuther Plan envisions comprehensive benefits, although these might be introduced in stages. Contrary to the other plans, the Reuther Plan acknowledges the need for reorganization of the health delivery system, but no concrete proposals have been advanced beyond the vague idea of "incentives" to encourage group practice, regional planning, cost controls, etc. The proposal that a billion dollars be creamed off the top of the first year's collections and allocated to solving delivery system problems appears to be no more than an afterthought. And many of the forms of reorganization of the delivery system envisioned, e.g., hospital-based group practices, seem to be motivated more by their cost-saving potential than by their implications for patient care.

Regardless of these shortcomings, the Reuther Plan has been dubbed the most progressive of the three types, and thereby has attracted the support of such health liberals as Michael DeBakey, M.D., heart specialist and originator of the regional medical programs; Mary Lasker, philanthropist who guided the development of the National Institutes of Health; and Whitney Young, director of the Urban League. The A.F.L.-C.I.O. plan, embodied in legislation introduced in Congress by Representative Martha Griffiths, is similar in most respects to the Reuther Plan.

Other proposals for national health insurance are being developed. Senator Javits is reported to be working with former Secretary of H.E.W. Wilbur Cohen (the architect of the Medicare program) on a proposal that will resemble Medicare. At this writing, it is uncertain how the Javits Plan will differ from the Reuther Plan. Recently, Senator Ted Kennedy made a statement sketching broad outlines for a national health insurance program that would be introduced in stages, similar to the Reuther Plan, but financed primarily through general tax revenues.

Liberal critics have seen major shortcomings in all of the plans so far advanced.

(1) All of the plans will reinforce the fee-for-service system. So long as doctors can choose to be reimbursed on a fee-for-service basis within a national health insurance system (despite the plans' "encouragement" toward prepaid group practice), this fragmented, inefficient, and costly form of delivering care will be preserved, and the political strength of the status quo-oriented doctors will be reinforced.

(2) All of the plans will leave the system dependent on private health insurance companies. Even the Reuther Plan, in which the government is the insurance company, will probably enlist Blue Cross to administer the plan.

(3) The national health insurance plans, as presently proposed, have come up with no workable and equitable mechanism for controlling costs, and will merely fuel the inflationary fire now consuming the health care system.

(4) Most of the proposals for national health insurance, including the labor-backed plans, are based on regressive methods of taxation. Flat rate, employee-employer payroll taxes take a bigger proportional bite out of the wages of low-paid workers than of high-paid workers.

(5) None of the plans makes any provision for significant consumer-community participation in program planning or in budgeting.

Many medical students and younger professionals, active in organizations such as the Medical Committee for Human Rights and the Student Health Organization, argue that these criticisms beg the question. No national health *insurance* system is going to solve the basic problems of the American health care system, they say.

National health insurance, to be sure, may well be a useful reform for many Americans. It may help a few people pay for medical services which they would otherwise not get. It may shore up a few hospitals in low-income areas whose total collapse would be a tragedy for the people of the community. It is hard to oppose a measure which, in however limited a way, may help a few people, at least, to have greater access to badly needed health services. But national health insurance, in the end, (1) won't work, and (2) will have regressive effects as well as progressive ones.

The problem is that national health insurance will be a mechanism to funnel money out of the pockets of workers and taxpayers into the hands of the people who now run (and misrun) the health service delivery system—the doctors, the hospital administrators, and the Medical-Industrial complex which fattens on people's illnesses. It will thus strengthen those forces that insist that all health care must center on the doctor and the hospital, rather than the forces who wish to totally reorganize the delivery of health care.

At the same time, national health insurance will throw a cloud over what is really happening. To liberals, for whom national health insurance has long been a goal, it will appear that the problems of the medical system are being solved. Middle-class doubts as to the organization of care may be allayed temporarily if part of the bill is paid by someone else. An aura of good will and liberalism will surround President Nixon. The accelerating movement for more fundamental reorganization of the medical care system will be defused, at least for a while.

Meanwhile, national health insurance will solve nothing. First, it is unlikely that any of the proposed plans will be very effective in meeting people's health needs. For this we have the evidence of Medicaid and Medicare. Medicaid, for example, clearly showed that giving the poor an unlimited credit card for medical service did not end the two-class system of medicine. There are other, non-financial stumbling blocks: institutional inaccessibility, the relationship between doctor and patient; the control by the doctors of priorities for allocating funds, time, and equipment among research, teaching, and patient care; and the unaccountability of the hospital to the medical needs of the community. Medical care is sold in a monopolistic, not a free market place. The effect of national health insurance, as with Medicaid and Medicare, may well be a sizeable number of individuals who are enabled to pay for better care. But it will not create and make accessible high quality medical services for the great majority of poor and middle-class people.

Second, the hopes of some of the insurance plan advocates that the medical care system can be reorganized through incentives linked to the insurance scheme's repayment system will almost certainly be dashed. For example, one plan has proposed giving hospitals incentives to operate efficiently. This might save money, but at best, it would have no effect on the patterns of care in the institutions, on the relations of the institution to the community, and on the quality of care. In fact, unless very stringent controls by the community were introduced, the probable result would be that the hospital would cut down on service in order to save money and pick up its incentive reward. For another thing, economic incentives can at best only conquer economic obstacles to change. They have no power over the other pillars of the two-class medical system. For example, economic incentives may encourage a hospital to be more economical, but they are unlikely to persuade a hospital to accept community control, or to convince $50,000-a-year doctors to put care of the indigent ahead of prestigious research. Finally, incentives are slow. We can't wait twenty or thirty years just to get doctors into group practices.

The third way in which national health insurance will fail will be economic. We have seen in the past few years how Medicaid and Medicare fed galloping medical inflation. The mechanisms are clear: the medical establishment which commanded the use of funds used them for their own priorities—prestigious and expensive and "interesting" medical technology, and high salaries for doctors and administrators. As a result, costs soared, while patient care improved only slightly, if at all. There is no reason to think the same thing would not be repeated under national health insurance. No workable cost control law has yet been devised, and, in any case, the impulse of hospital administrators is to cut costs at the expense of patients and hospital workers. It is entirely conceivable that in 1975, under national health insurance, the nation will be spending $90 billion a year instead of the present $60 billion for health services, and $200 a day for a hospital bed, without any significant improvement in the quality of care for the average citizen.

National health insurance will fail because it fails to face the fundamental questions about our health system—control, accountability, accessibility, priorities, responsibility to the community. And it fails this test precisely because it is national health *insurance*. Under an insurance mechanism, no matter how liberal, the private delivery system performs a certain service and the public funding (insurance) system pays for it. The public insurers may try to persuade the controllers of the private delivery system to change the system, but no attempt is made to take the power to control away from them. The key issues about the health system are thus removed from the discussion right from the start.

To this dead end, we can only propose the fundamental alternatives: the only way to fundamentally change the health system so that it provides adequate, dignified care for all is to take power over health care away from the people who now control it. Not merely the funding of the health system, but the system itself must be public. It then becomes possible to face such questions as how such a "national health *system*" can be made responsive to the community and accountable to it, how to insure that patient care is the primary priority of the system, how to insure equal access to health institutions and to practitioners, and so on.

Many people have suggested that national health insurance might be a step toward such a national health system. Others argue it will be regressive. By providing financing, it will stave off the collapse of the present system for a few short years, and will strengthen some of the enemies of change. At the same time, though, it will establish the necessity for the government to guarantee the right to health care for all, and it will arouse even greater expectations of adequate health care. Thus national health insurance is not clearly either a step towards or a step away from a national health system—it's more of a shuffle sideways.

XIII

THE BEST-LAID PLANS . . .

Like other sectors of the American economy, the health industry is, at least formally, "unplanned." Until quite recently, the absence of planning was not seen as a serious flaw in the industry. It was assumed for health, as for other industries, that the laws of the marketplace would automatically keep things running smoothly—matching supply to demand and prices to wages. Planning was not only unnecessary, it was counter to the spirit of a free society. But over the last ten years, the realization has deepened that the laws of the marketplace can just as easily work to produce absolute scarcity, mounting demand, and orbiting prices. Even the most enthusiastic advocates of medical free enterprise have had to admit that the unbridled self-interests of health financing and health care institutions do not add up to a rational health system. With some rhetorical reluctance, captains of the health service industry have gradually added planning to their armory of skills.

We all know that the health industry has never really been unplanned. Every year hospitals are built, insurance plans sold, doctors graduated—all achievements which require years of foresight, in fact, of planning. Just the existence of thousands of health facilities buildings (often very old) testifies to the fact that planning of some kind has been going on for decades. Further, the existence of administratively-linked networks of facilities—medical empires (see chapters III through V)—suggests that even what we now call regional planning has been quietly occurring for the last decade. This kind of planning, the kind of planning which results in buildings, is never acclaimed, in fact, rarely even announced. It occurs quietly and privately, over gala fund-raising dinners and intimate lunches, in the faculty clubs of medical schools, in private clubs, at board meetings of philanthropic agencies and hospitals. Participation is by invitation only, and does not extend beyond the men who control existing health facilities—trustees and directors of hospitals, deans of medical schools, philanthropists and health insurance executives.

The last decade has seen superficially striking changes in the style, though rarely the substance, of health planning. The planners by and large remain the same. But the means by which they interact, negotiate and put forth their decisions have been increasingly formalized. The areawide health planning movement, as it is called, began as a nationwide phenomenon in the late fifties and picked up steam through state and federal sanction in the early sixties, until by 1966, there were a total of eighty areawide health planning agencies around the country. To farsighted medical liberals of the early sixties, these planning agencies represented a safe compromise between the values of a free enterprise system and the need for firm planning to curb rising disorganization in the health system. The local areawide planning agencies were voluntary (i.e., under private, nonprofit auspices) rather than government sponsored, but they always had considerable force of persuasion and they often had some force of law.

Prime instigators of the areawide health planning movement were the financiers of hospital care and hospital construction—Blue Cross, philanthropic organizations, commercial insurance companies, and representatives of large-scale employers. Hospital operating and construction costs had already begun their twenty-year race with the consumer price index, and the financiers of care hoped to either cut costs or reduce the public's use of hospitals. Since cost cutting would have run into organized resistance from the hospitals, the financiers of care concentrated on trying to limit the use of hospitals, largely by limiting the construction of new hospitals. Professionally staffed, "scientific," and "broadly representative" planning agencies, set up with the task of reviewing plans for new hospital construction, served to justify unpopular, bed-limiting planning decisions. Initially funded privately —by Blue Cross in Michigan, the steel industry in Pittsburgh, philanthropic organizations and Blue Cross in New York City—many of these agencies gradually won public financing and authority, although they remained privately run and publicly unaccountable.

On their own terms, many of the nation's areawide health facility planning agencies were solidly successful. The best attracted impressive professional planning staffs and won the enthusiastic participation of the local hospitals. Hospitals, no less than hospital financiers, were concerned lest new hospitals lure away their patients (empty beds are almost as expensive to maintain as full ones, and, of course, are not paid for by patients). Even expansionist hospitals were, by the sixties, too dependent on Blue Cross and the other third party plans to ignore the local areawide health facilities planning agency. The paragon among the nation's areawide planning agencies is New York City's Health and Hospital Planning Council, which brings together business, health insurers, a few trade unions, philanthropies, and all the city's medical empires. The success of this elite coalition can be measured in terms of the number of hospital beds which would have been built in New York if it hadn't been for the Council: New York City now has a persistent and dangerous shortage of hospital beds.

The federal government was apparently content with the efforts of the nation's scattered areawide planning agencies until 1966, when it, too, became a major health care financier. With Medicaid and Medicare, the Johnson administration felt it had guaranteed payment for health care to almost all Americans. Its only remaining concern was to guarantee the existence of high quality sources of care for the new Medicaid and Medicare cardholders. Federally financed neighborhood health centers represented one part of this effort, but, by and large, the government preferred to limit itself to stimulating the private sector in health to meet the new demand. The results were the Regional Medical Program (R.M.P., Public Law 89-239) and the Comprehensive Health Planning legislation (C.H.P., Public Law 89-749) of 1966. Both were attempts to promote *positive* planning, that is, planning to meet people's needs, rather than to put a check on hospitals' capital decisions. Both were widely heralded, both from the left and the medical moderates, as programs with potentially far greater impact than either Medicaid or Medicare—programs which would truly make high quality care a right for all while at the same time rationalizing and streamlining the health care delivery system.

With neither R.M.P. or C.H.P. was the federal government attempting to bypass or supersede existing voluntary planning mechanisms. The idea was to build on and broaden the established planning mechanisms where they existed, and to create new ones where they did not. C.H.P.

aimed to create regional planning agencies throughout the nation, patterned after New York's Health and Hospital Planning Council, but concerned with medical services, environmental health, manpower, etc., as well as construction—and run with greater input from health care consumers. R.M.P. was to stimulate regional cooperative arrangements between medical schools and to encourage the schools to plan for more effective translation of medical discoveries into medical practice, focusing on the killer diseases, heart disease, cancer and stroke.

Today, four years after the birth of R.M.P. and C.H.P. the health care delivery system is no more rational and integrated than it was in 1966. Health services have not become a right guaranteed by one's Blue Cross, Medicaid or Medicare card, but are still a prize, won from the providers of care only by the most skillful, patient-consumers. These planning programs, which looked so obvious and rational from the sweeping vantage point of national health policy, have simply failed to take root in the hard ground of local health politics. Only a handful of Comprehensive Health Planning Agencies have sprung up across the nation, and many of them are the already existing planning agencies, spruced up with the rhetoric of comprehensiveness and representativeness. In most other areas which have so far merited C.H.P. funds, the recipient is an agency set up to *plan* a Comprehensive Health Planning Agency. R.M.P. agencies are more widespread, but have given up on their original missions of planning and regionalization and become little more than funding sources for medical schools' pet projects. It was hardly a surprise, even to federal R.M.P. and C.H.P. staff, when the Nixon administration began in late 1969 to mutter about phasing out the two programs.

Even with aggressive federal backing, it is not clear that R.M.P. and C.H.P. could have lived up to their radical promise. The programs were charged with the task of creating an excellent and rational American health system, but they were not given the authority to require a single institution to alter its plans or policies in the smallest detail. There is nothing in the R.M.P. legislation which explains how the program will deal with medical schools which are not interested in cooperative arrangements. And there is not a line in the C.H.P. legislation which tells how local comprehensive planning agencies will be empowered to implement their plans. The federal government's ability to force change rested in the twenty or so billion dollars it invested in Medicaid and Medicare, and this money flowed out through channels independent of R.M.P. and C.H.P.—free from any planning or reorganizational constraints. R.M.P. and C.H.P. were never designed to create effective, public planning mechanisms. They were designed to gently stimulate local private health establishments to take, in the course of their usual planning, some account of the needs of the public.

If R.M.P. and C.H.P. are, through various stages of underfinancing and bureaucratic shuffling, phased out of existence, they will go with hardly a whimper. Medical schools may regret the passing of R.M.P. and its ready store of petty cash, and many health planning agencies will miss the glamor of C.H.P., but most health financing and providing institutions will be just as happy to revert to or stick with their traditional styles of planning. Very few, if any, health consumers will put up a fuss, since most of them understood long ago that the new federal programs were, at best, new names for the same old elite planning processes and, at worst, instruments for the further consolidation of the forces which now control local health systems. For instance, to the extent that medical schools have chosen to use it, R.M.P.'s mandate for regionalization has promoted the consolidation and centralization of existing medical empires. C.H.P., where it has gotten off the ground at all, has strengthened existing elite planning mechanisms, and given them a liberal lustre. Whether it was the areawide planning movement of the early sixties or the more avant-garde Federal planning programs of the mid-sixties, efforts to rationalize the American health system have only succeeded in strengthening the grip of the socially irrational forces which already determine who will be cared for, how, and at what price.

XIV

COMPREHENSIVE HEALTH PLANNING:

CONFRONTATION OVER THE

DRAWING BOARDS

Health-facilities-planning was the health fad of the sixties. Local health planning agencies sprang up all over the country; universities began to offer Ph.D. programs in health planning; and the federal government set up a bureaucracy and a budget to support local planning efforts. Asked to define "planning" and illustrate its accomplishments, partisans of the health facilities planning movement point with pride to a single agency, New York City's Health and Hospital Planning Council (H.H.P.C.), renowned throughout the nation as the prototypical health facilities planning agency. Established in the thirties, H.H.P.C. set the pattern for the scores of planning agencies which sprang up in the early sixties: it limited its planning to maintaining a veto over decisions to build or rebuild facilities (i.e., it was a "facilities" planning agency, rather than a "comprehensive" planning agency); it was privately controlled, although increasingly publicly funded; it was dominated by local hospitals and Blue Cross. By the mid-sixties, major cities such as Detroit, Pittsburgh, Cleveland, and Toledo each boasted a planning agency modeled after H.H.P.C. In 1966, when the federal government moved to stimulate a national program of health planning, Secretary of H.E.W. Wilbur Cohen, in his testimony to a Senate committee, cited H.H.P.C. as a model of regional health planning. Congressman Staggers, in his report to the House on the new federal Comprehensive Health Planning (C.H.P.) Act of 1966, stated that the purpose of the act was "to extend and expand" existing private areawide planning efforts, such as H.H.P.C.

Today, four years later, the health planning movement nationally has begun to lose momentum, and in New York City, H.H.P.C. itself has begun to lose some of its delusions of grandeur. In 1967, in the words of its annual report, H.H.P.C. saw itself as "free from the pressures of political expediency yet sensitive to the needs and desires of local groups,"and possessing "wisdom and courage in making the hard planning decisions." Now repeated attacks by ghetto community organizations have smashed H.H.P.C.'s image as an evenhanded arbiter of the health needs of the city, and discredited it as a tool of the private medical empires and Blue Cross. Nationwide, the new Comprehensive Health Planning effort shows signs of being as bankrupt as the model on which it was based. Comprehensive Health Planning has either failed to take hold —wrecked by the resistance of existing agencies like H.H.P.C.—or, worse, has served to strengthen the grip of the old planning agencies and the powerful private institutions which they represent.

Health and Hospital Planning Council, like Blue Cross, was a child of the Depression. The Depression brought financial disaster to the voluntary hospitals as the poor crowded into the municipal hospitals, leaving thousands of empty private beds in the voluntaries. In its efforts to en-

sure the economic wellbeing of the voluntaries, the United
Hospital Fund, then as now the leading institution of the
New York voluntary hospital establishment, formed the
Hospital Council (which has since become H.H.P.C.) and
a local Blue Cross plan. Blue Cross was to ensure that there
were enough paying patients. The Hospital Council was
to ensure that there weren't too many beds.

Despite the Depression there was a 6.6 percent increase
in hospital beds in New York City between 1930 and 1935.
This terrified most of the voluntaries; they had visions of
losing their increasingly rare paying patients to the hospitals with newer facilities. They were also worried that the
municipal hospitals, with an occupancy rate of 97.2 percent
(compared to 68.8 percent for the voluntaries), would expand and further draw patients away from the voluntary
system. So the Hospital Council was formed in 1934 as an
unincorporated voluntary association "to develop a coordinated hospital program for the city." The Council took
it upon itself to review all proposals for hospital construction with the criteria that no hospital project be launched
"unless it can be shown to be necessary, timely, reasonably
assured of support and wisely located."

In 1937 the Hospital Survey, a study initiated by the
United Hospital Fund, recommended that a "permanent,
representative and authoritative" central planning and
coordinating body be established to save the community
from the "extravagance and waste in hospital building and
maintenance." Its prestige enhanced by the recommendations of the Hospital Survey, the Hospital Council incorpo-
rated in 1938. Its only power to enforce its planning
decisions was its ability to persuade benefactors of hospitals to withhold financial support from unapproved programs. In 1947 it got considerably more power when, as the

regional agent for the federal Hill-Burton hospital construction program, it became itself a hospital benefactor. Between 1948 and 1963 it determined how over twenty-one million dollars of hospital construction funds were spent in the city.

The financial distress of Blue Cross in the late fifties and early sixties gave the planning movement in general and H.H.P.C. in particular a big boost. Increases in the cost of hospital care and in the utilization of hospitals threatened to bankrupt Blue Cross and its dependents, the voluntary hospitals. Up until the late '50s Blue Cross had been able to pass its cost increases on to its subscribers. Between 1945 and 1963 Blue Cross in New York State increased its group rates for family coverage by 453 to 708 percent. By the late '50s state insurance officials charged with regulating Blue Cross began to resist approving Blue Cross' never-ending applications for rate increases, sometimes to the point of actually refusing them. Caught in the bind between increasing costs and the increasing resistance of state officials, and threatened by competitive private insurance companies who offered cash benefits rather than service benefits, Blue Cross turned to regional planning as a way to control its costs.

But regional health planning meant little more to Blue Cross than stopping the construction of any new hospital beds or, better still, reducing the number of beds. Hospital utilization is directly related to bed availability; if there are fewer beds, fewer people can be filling them, and Blue Cross' maximum liabiity is reduced. Restricting the number of beds also leads to optimal occupancy rates for the existing hospitals, so, by and large, the hospitals' interests were met, too.

In some states, such as Michigan, Blue Cross moved to

enforce its planning by refusing to reimburse hospitals that had been constructed without its approval. In New York, Blue Cross lobbied successfully for laws that gave authority to regional planning agencies to review all hospital construction and renovation. The Hospital Council, more fashionably renamed the Hospital Reviewing and Planning Council (and still later, the Health and Hospital Planning Council), was given this authority in 1964 for the New York City area. Although final authority to approve or disapprove hospital construction rests in the state Department of Health, the state rarely reverses the Council's decisions.

To ensure that the Council had enough money to function "properly" under the new laws, New York City Blue Cross increased its annual support of the Council from $10,000 to $100,000. In 1968 the Council received over two-thirds of its private (nongovernment) support from Blue Cross, the United Hospital Fund, and the Greater New York Fund (whose health donations are distributed by the United Hospital Fund). Support from religious and labor groups amounted to less than ten percent of the amount given by Blue Cross and the United Hospital Fund. Altogether, the private support makes up only about a quarter of the total budget; the rest comes from the state and federal governments.

Even within the H.H.P.C. some have questioned the role of Blue Cross in health planning agencies. George Baehr, who is on the Board of Directors of the Health and Hospital Planning Council warned in a September, 1968, letter to the President of H.H.P.C., "At the instigation of the Blue Cross plans, Hospital Review and Planning Councils in several states are now endeavoring to persuade state and local governmental authorities to deny approval for the construction of any additional hospital beds so that the number in their area may be kept to an irreducible minimum, and thereby 'put the squeeze' on the medical profession. The existence of an excessive number of hospital beds in a community unquestionably encourages overutilization. On the other hand, if controls are carried too far in an effort to keep down Blue Cross insurance rates through the device of bed scarcity, a serious public health hazard may be created."

In New York City, the Council's policy of limiting hospital construction has been an unqualified success: it has already produced a public health hazard. *The New York Times* has recently reported that the voluntary hospitals are crowded to the crisis point. Some are now operating at an occupancy rate of ninety-five percent, far in excess of the eighty to eighty-five percent occupancy rate that most administrators consider wise. A man in imminent danger of losing his life usually can get a bed somewhere but often it is a second- or third-rate hospital instead of the well-equipped, well-staffed one where he would have the best chance of survival. It is probably the proprietary (profit-making) hospitals which have benefited the most from the Council's bed-limiting policy. They are now operating at eighty-six percent of capacity, whereas, as recently as 1960, they were operating at seventy-one percent of capacity.

For all practical purposes, H.H.P.C. has stopped pretending to do objective health planning and has openly become the voluntary hospitals' apologist. Best-known is the case of St. Francis Hospital, in the heart of the south Bronx's health desert, which was serving a population becoming increasingly poor and nonwhite. In 1965 the Archdiocese of New York decided it wanted to close St.

Francis. Having run $500,000 into the red in 1964, St. Francis was proving to be too much of a drain on the Archdiocese's resources. So the Council was asked to review the situation. The Council had previously thought favorably of St. Francis and stressed the need for it. In fact, it called a modernization and expansion planned for St. Francis a "welcome development." However, in response to the prodding of the Archdiocese, the Council in 1965 decided that it was "impractical for St. Francis Hospital to continue operation as a voluntary general hospital care facility in the South Bronx" and recommended that the hospital "cease operations as soon as practicable." In the uproar that followed, the Archdiocese changed its mind. The Council promptly reversed its recommendation, too. In October 1966, the Council was to reverse itself once more. The Archidocese withdrew its support for a new St. Francis, and in response the Council decided once again that there was no need in the South Bronx for a new St. Francis.

The Bronx Morrisania Hospital caper is an illustration of the Council's role as an *ex post facto* apologist for medical empire builders. Public and private healer-dealers had worked out a grand scheme for the Bronx. The voluntary health establishment would allow a new hospital to be built in a decaying neighborhood of the West Bronx provided that Morrisania Hospital (a municipal hospital now located in a poverty area) be relocated in the hospital-rich northwest Bronx. The Council was then called in for its recommendations. In January 1968 the Council approved the plan, even though it was in direct contradiction to the results of the Council's most recent study of the Bronx, dated December 1966. In this study it was concluded that it was not possible at this time to choose an optimum site for a new Morrisania Hospital due to continuing shifts in population and hospitalization patterns in the Bronx. Presumably to protect its credibility, the Council suppressed the Bronx report, after only limited circulation.

Through the St. Francis incident, and H.H.P.C.'s simultaneous protracted opposition to a new hospital for Manhattan's densely populated lower east side ghetto (see chapter XIX), H.H.P.C. had won for itself a degree of community resentment normally reserved for more visible, front-line health agencies. Thus the 1966 discussions of a new comprehensive health planning agency found in New York City an alert and sophisticated audience. The new agency, to be federally financed through 1966 legislation (PL 89-749), was to be concerned with much more than construction and destruction of beds. It would have positive planning power over physical facilities, service programs, and manpower for medical, mental health, and environmental services. According to the federal law, these comprehensive powers would be vested in a single regional agency representing a partnership of consumers, providers and public officials. The law's most radical feature was the requirement that this partnership be composed of a majority of health service consumers.

H.H.P.C. had every reason to expect that, as New York City's seasoned and authoritative health planning agency, it would be designated as the "new" Comprehensive Planning Agency—a fitting accolade for so many years of voluntary service. In 1966, H.H.P.C. smugly began preparations for its transformation into a Comprehensive Health Planning Agency. It was at this time that the name was changed from Hospital Planning and Review Council, with the word "health" thrown in to acknowledge its widening sphere of concern. At the same time, H.H.P.C.

added an established, consumer-oriented private welfare
agency to its roster of member organizations—so that the
transition to a consumer majority could take place without
disrupting the existing balance of power. With this face-
lifting accomplished, H.H.P.C. was ready, in 1967, to sit
down with city health officials and negotiate for city approval of its bid for comprehensive health planning powers, a necessary prerequisite to the presentation of a formal
proposal to the state government.

Community leadership in Harlem, the Bronx, and the
lower east side was enraged when the news of H.H.P.C.'s
quiet preparations broke. In what was probably the nation's first organized attack on anything as arcane as a
health facilities planning agency, a coalition of community
groups staged a demonstration outside of H.H.P.C.'s fashionable Fifth Avenue headquarters. The coalition continued to grow throughout 1968, arguing, chiefly through
leaflets to the communities and petitions to the Mayor, for
a *public* agency to be given comprehensive health planning powers. Some of the opposition went further, assert-
ing that a partnership of providers and consumers would
never work out—planning powers should be vested in a
neighborhood-based, all-consumer organization. As Victor
Solomon, 1968 Chairman of Harlem CORE put it, "You
can't put a rat, a cat, and a dog in one room and expect
them to come out agreeing on anything."

Under pressure from the city's first organized, citywide
coalition of neighborhood health groups, Mayor Lindsay
unexpectedly announced that the city would enter the lists
with its own proposal for a public comprehensive planning
agency. H.H.P.C. was justifiably chagrined, for the city
health officialdom had never been anything but cooperative in the past. And if the city's bid won, H.H.P.C. would

be out of a job, losing all its existing federal funds and its functions to the new planning agency.

Even more unexpected to H.H.P.C. than the city's betrayal was the Brutus-like behavior of many of H.H.P.C.'s own private hospital and philanthropic agencies, who put up only token defense of H.H.P.C. Many agencies had found that they could not rely on H.H.P.C. for routine planning data, much less for long-term considerations. Some of New York City's more technocratically oriented private sector spokesmen had long since given up on H.H.P.C. as a rational and scientific planning agency. Many of the others, unperturbed by H.H.P.C.'s technical failings, were simply impressed by the fact that H.H.P.C. had been universally discredited as a scientific planning agency, and would no longer serve as an acceptable front for private decisions.

With its private sector support eroding, even the marked favoritism of the state authorities was not enough to guarantee H.H.P.C. a victory over the city. For months the state procrastinated, alternately rejecting both city and H.H.P.C. proposals as insufficiently demonstrative of a true "partnership." The final outcome was in itself a procrastination; the city was granted authority to set up an agency to plan for a comprehensive planning agency. For the two-year period while the planning-to-plan agency plans a comprehensive health planning agency, H.H.P.C. will continue business as usual. In a 1969 letter to the city's chief health officer, the president of H.H.P.C. announced that the city's partial victory "does not alter the present commitments and responsibilities of the Health and Hospital Planning Council of Southern New York, Inc." H.H.P.C., with ample representation on the City's planning-to-plan agency, has two years to reassert itself as *the*

New York City health planning agency.

Across the country, the story of local efforts at health planning has many parallels to the case of H.H.P.C. in New York City. Where the private institutional forces in health—Blue Cross, voluntary health and welfare agencies, medical school-hospital empires—are strong and well-organized, voluntary health planning agencies have thrived, and have served their masters well. In the medical empire-dominated urban centers, comprehensive health planning has meant, at best, some reshuffling of the forces already involved in health planning, and, at worst, a re-naming of the old health planning agencies. In rural areas, with more primitive, doctor-centered health care systems, formal health planning was rarely contemplated until the advent of Comprehensive Health Planning (C.H.P.). In such areas, particularly in the south and southwest, the task of implementing C.H.P. has fallen largely to county health officers, drawing on local medical societies for representation of medical care providers (doctors and hospitals).

Some of the C.H.P.-sparked reshuffling has been catac-lysmic enough to strike fear into the hearts of entrenched voluntary planning agencies and their constituent private health institutions. New York is not the only city where C.H.P. provoked a confrontation between local public health authorities and an established voluntary planning agency. In Cleveland, for instance, Mayor Stokes refused to approve the local planning voluntary council's applica-tion for C.H.P. funds, and won, like Mayor Lindsay in New York, a two-year preplanning breathing spell. Im-pressed by such cases, nationally prominent health econo-mist (and voluntary hospital apologist) Ann Somers, wrote in the August, 1969, issue of the *Journal of the American Hospital Association* , "Passage of PL 89-749 [C.H.P.] confused the entire situation . . . it has, perhaps unknowingly, tended to undermine the essential institutional base for health care planning—the hospital." Even more alarmed, an executive of the Ohio Hospital Association said in an October, 1968, meeting sponsored by the American Hospital Association, that existing voluntary planning agencies "are in jeopardy of continuing to function effectively, if at all." New York's H.H.P.C., in its 1967-68 annual report, complained:

> Unfortunately, however, Public Law 89-749 has already confused the health planning process in many local communities, particularly in those areas where existing areawide health facility planning agencies are competing with local health departments, county medical societies, civic planning authorities, or other community groups for recognition as the local comprehensive health planning body . . . just when many such agencies were forging ahead, despite serious obstacles, in solving many pressing health and hospital problems of their communities this new element of competition is introduced.

The fears of hospital associations and health planning agencies are gradually subsiding, however. As C.H.P. inches ahead across the nation, it is becoming clear that the worst the established planning agencies have to look forward to is simply confusion, and that probably only temporarily. In city after city, the old planning agencies are working out a variety of ingenious accommodations with the uncompetitive competition posed by C.H.P. By far the most common, in fact, *the* method of choice in over 90 percent of the areas now receiving any federal funds through C.H.P., is the route taken in Cleveland and New York—the postponement of the creation of an official C.H.P. agency during a two-year organizational or preplanning period. This gives the old facilities-planning agency a period of grace to consolidate its strength, and, at the same time, an opportunity to play an important role in the preplanning agency. When the preplanning phase is over, the old facilities-planning agency can then follow the example of its counterparts in areas which already have fully operative C.H.P. agencies. It can beef itself up to become the C.H.P. agency; it can push for the new C.H.P. agency to become an umbrella organization with itself as the member organization assigned to do facilities planning; or, at worst, it can acquiesce to the creation of a new agency to do comprehensive health planning, then do all the facilities planning under subcontract to the new agency. In either case, the existing planning agency retains its grip over facilities planning—and hence over the ultimate distribution of medical resouces in the region.

Where C.H.P. agencies, or preplanning agencies, have gotten started, they have made little change in the traditional health planning process. What was supposed to be new about comprehensive health planning was not just the name of the agency in charge. C.H.P. was to depart from traditional, elite-dominated, facility-centered health planning in two respects: C.H.P. agencies were to be headed up by boards consisting of a majority of health services consumers, and they were to be concerned with health in the broadest sense, including environmental and preventive factors. Nationwide, the best known failure of local C.H.P. efforts is their staunch, and often ingenious, exclusion of any new consumer faces. A leading H.E.W. bureaucrat admitted to a group of low-income neighborhood representatives in late 1969 that a consumer is usually defined for C.H.P. purposes as "a local doctor's wife, a retired doctor or hospital trustee," and the federal government is powerless to stop these violations of the spirit of the legislation. Hospitals and health care financers are, of course, delighted with local C.H.P.'s broad notion of "consumers." The Health Insurance Council, the national association of commercial health insurance companies, boasts that the insurance industry has representatives on half the nation's C.H.P. preplanning or operative agencies, all of them listed as "consumers." And most voluntary hospital associations would agree with the administrator of Baylor University Medical Center in Dallas when he listed, as qualifications of consumers to be involved in health planning: "education, leadership ability, a broad sense of civic responsibility, and experience in making decisions affecting the welfare of people and expenditure of large sums of money." Hence the overwhelming representation of local business leaders—often hospital trustees in their spare time—on C.H.P. agencies. So systematic has been the exclusion of poor and working-class consumers from comprehensive health planning boards that one regional division of H.E.W. was driven, in 1969, to produce a long and plaintive document entitled "Why and How to Involve People of Disadvantaged Circumstances in Governing Boards of Comprehensive Health Planning Agencies."

Comprehensiveness, no more than representativeness, has not been an outstanding quality of C.H.P. efforts to date. In a 1969 survey of C.H.P. agencies (both preplanning and operational), the great majority listed as their primary concern facilities planning, with manpower, environment, and services for the poor and aged running well behind. This fascination with bricks and mortar was as prevalent among new agencies as among those which had been facilities-planning agencies—probably indicating the sizeable influence of the old facilities-planning agencies over supposedly new C.H.P. agencies. Of course, C.H.P. agencies have not been single-mindedly involved in facilities construction. Among the enterprises listed in an August, 1969, study performed by the American Rehabilitative Foundation of C.H.P. agencies around the country as major achievements in 1968 were such things as, "prepared an Orientation Booklet . . . ," "promoted local millage [taxation] for county health departments," and "worked with civil defense agency to upgrade emergency plans."

But, after all, what does it matter? Formal health planning in the United States has always been voluntary, both in terms of who controlled it and how it was implemented. (New York and the few other states which added legal muscle to the authority of voluntary health facilities planning agencies were exceptional.) All the indications are that comprehensive health planning will be far more peripheral, more powerless than the old voluntary facilities planning. The federal law says nothing about how local comprehensive health plans are to be implemented, and the states have been just as indefinite. (In New York, for instance, there is no state law providing for new C.H.P. agencies to take over the powers now vested by the state in voluntary planning agencies.) The interpretation of C.H.P. current in government as well as private circles is that C.H.P. agencies will have no more than an advisory role with respect to the plans of private health institutions. For instance, H.E.W. official James Cavanaugh wrote in the November, 1969, issue of the *Journal of the American Hospital Association*,

> . . . planning is not a final decision-making process but is instead, a process of projecting, documenting and recommending alternatives in order to present decision-makers with a set of choices.

Needless to say, the American Hospital Association in its 1969 "Statement on Financial Requirements of Health Care Institutions and Services" agreed that "the primary function of [a C.H.P. agency] is to serve regularly in the capacity of adviser and consultant. . . ." C.H.P. staff directors show no signs of stepping out of line. In the survey cited before, the majority listed their functions as "advisory," "serving as a data source," and "coordination." C.H.P., once seen as a means of rationalizing and democratizing health planning, has thus become just another public subsidy of the privately-managed and privately-planned American health and hospital system.

XV

REGIONAL MEDICAL PROGRAMS:
MEDICAL SCHOOLS ON THE MAKE

Of the many contradictions in American medicine, none is more ironic than the contrast between the promise of biomedical technology and the tawdry reality of medical care. Major centers of medical research and education, such as Harvard Medical Center, Johns Hopkins, and Columbia, abut on urban slums, which are some of the nation's most disgraceful backwaters of medical neglect. Outside of the big cities, with their occasional medical centers of excellence, there are the hundreds and thousands of smaller cities and suburban regions, whose small, isolated medical facilities practice the medicine which was taught twenty years ago. The high technology of medicine filters only slowly, almost accidentally, down from the centers of excellence where it is generated to the outposts of mediocrity where it is applied to human care.

Bridging the gap between the production and distribution of medical technology was a major priority of the Kennedy-Johnson "Health New Deal" of the sixties. Comprehensive Health Planning was to make the health care delivery system function more rationally and equitably; the Regional Medical Program (R.M.P.) was to bring the fruits of science to the health care delivery system.

Through R.M.P., medical excellence would be decentralized from the current handful of major medical centers to a whole network of little pockets of excellence, all under the general guidance of the major medical centers. Through the R.M.P. network, technological advances would flow swiftly from the medical school laboratory to the suburban hospital or rural doctor's office. Emphasis at both the research and delivery ends of this system was to be on heart, cancer, and stroke, the diseases which drag down American life-expectancy figures to levels below those for a dozen or more other nations. Since most people, including congressmen, are worried about heart disease, cancer, and stroke, R.M.P. seemed bound to start out with a natural constituency of millions.

R.M.P. was the brainchild of a commission appointed in 1964 by President Johnson "to recommend steps to reduce the incidence of these diseases [heart disease, cancer, and stroke] through new knowledge and more complete utilization of the medical knowledge we already have." The commission, headed by heart surgeon Michael De Bakey, called for what would have been the farthest-reaching reforms in American medical history. At the delivery level, the commission called for the creation of a national network of centers where research could be directly integrated with patient care. Altogether sixty such centers were to be erected around the nation, and these sixty were to be ringed by 450 outposts for emergency and outpatient care and 100 units for rehabilitation services. Bolstering this new system for delivering care, there would be a massive expansion of medical research and education. The commission also called for the creation of twenty-five new biomedical research institutes throughout the country, and for direct federal support of medical education.

In itself, the De Bakey commission's report stands as the first example of a major systems-analysis and planning effort ever to be applied to the American medical system. In its recommendations, it came closer to calling for what the A.M.A. termed "socialized medicine" than any other health reform of the sixties, including Medicare and Medicaid. The federal government was already in the business of medical research. The De Bakey commission called for a direct federal role in what are still private property—patient care and medical education. The government would not only operate a vast new network of medical research and care facilities, it would use these to reshape the entire medical delivery system. Equally revolutionary was the call for the government to underwrite medical education—long underfinanced, at A.M.A. insistence, to limit the nation's supply of doctors.

It almost goes without saying that the De Bakey commission represented only a narrow element of the nation's medical establishment. Notably absent from membership were the A.M.A., the American Hospital Association, Blue Cross, and Blue Shield—the major organized forces in American health politics. What the commission represented was the more progressive, service-oriented segment of the nation's medical school elite, with a few corporate executives thrown in for good measure. The nation's medical schools as a whole, organized into the American Association of Medical Colleges (A.A.M.C.), are divided into two camps: the ivory tower patricians and the more service-oriented liberals. The philosophy of the former group is summed up in a 1953 report of the A.A.M.C., which warned medical schools against "building up large empires which serve as welfare and semicharitable institutions, steadily spreading their influence and control over many segments of health care." The expansionist liberal view, summed up in the Coggeshall Report of 1965, declared that the medical schools "should be appraising the needs of society for health care and health personnel," and "developing and implementing plans to meet these needs." In its philosophy, the De Bakey commission spoke for only the latter group, the medical school liberals who were interested in reorganizing the medical system with the medical schools at its center.

In the narrowest sense, even the most isolationist medical schools stood to gain a great deal from the De Bakey commission's plan. Direct federal support of medical research would take much of the anxiety and uncertainty out of research, by making federal support cover the entire cost of a research project (rather than leaving part of the bill for the medical school to pick up) and by greatly lengthening the allowable period of investigation for each research project. Thus, in return for their new responsibilities for promoting health care, the medical schools would gain a lasting subsidy for their internal activities.

But if the De Bakey commission stood for the medical schools, and especially for the more expansionist and liberal among them, the Regional Medical Program which finally emerged from Congress spoke for everyone the De Bakey commission had left out. First H.E.W. took over the commission report and translated it into a bill—minus the section on expanding medical education. The Johnson administration had just undertaken, through Medicare, to finance medical care for twenty million people, and it was not about to simultaneously take on the burden of subsidizing medical education, at least not while the Vietnam War was picking up momentum. What was left of the De Bakey report in the bill submitted by H.E.W. to the eighty-ninth

Congress won the instant support of the American Cancer Society, the American Hospital Association, and the American Association of Medical Colleges. That left only the A.M.A.

A.M.A. opposition centered on the bill's provision for a network of regional medical centers. Medicare had been bad enough, but this was socialized medicine! In late 1965, the president of the A.M.A., Dr. James Appel, said (according to the A.M.A. news release of Sept. 2, 1965): "Most medical leaders felt that the establishment of the series of medical complexes initially conceived [by the De Bakey Commission] would have had a more serious longterm effect on medical practice than the recently enacted Medicare law."

The A.M.A. then sat down with President Johnson and H.E.W. Secretary John Gardner to bargain: if the administration didn't change the R.M.P. bill to meet A.M.A. specifications, the A.M.A. would not cooperate with the new Medicare program, for which regulations were just being drawn up. The A.M.A. had its way. Twenty amendments were added to the Regional Medical Programs bill, which, Dr. Appel wrote, "will allay many of the fears the medical profession had about the original bill." Apparently not all the fears were allayed, for the A.M.A. still withheld its support from what was now, in large measure, its own bill.

The legislation, as finally enacted in 1966, was emasculated beyond recognition. Only one of the original recommendations of the commission had survived, probably because it was the vaguest, calling for

> grants to encourage and assist in the establishment of regional cooperative arrangements among medical schools, research institutions, and hospitals for research and training (including continuing education) and for related demonstrations of pa-

tient care in the fields of heart disease, cancer, stroke and related diseases.

Even this limited program carried the restriction that it was to be accomplished "without interfering with the patterns, or the methods of financing of patient care or professional practice, or with the administration of hospitals. . . ." The bill explicitly precluded any federal construction or operation of any regional heart disease, cancer, and stroke centers.

Conceived as a sweeping reorganization of the American medical system, R.M.P. had become a diffuse invitation to the nation's medical schools to take some responsibility for patient care, largely at the level of planning. Operationally, the law called on medical schools to organize voluntarily on a geographical basis, into "regional cooperative arrangements" linking the schools with hospitals and lesser health facilities. Everything hinged on these regional cooperative arrangements which were, hopefully, to be the means by which technological advances would be translated into patient care, and health facilities generally would come to partake of the excellence of the major medical school centers. All these changes were to be superimposed on the existing medical system as gently as possible. The congressional committee which acted on R.M.P. put it this way its formal report on the bill:

> The committee has been very careful to establish machinery in the bill which will insure local control of the programs conducted under the bill. The committee wishes to emphasize that this legislation is intended to be administered in such a way as to make no change whatsoever in the traditional methods of furnishing medical care to patients in the United States, or to financing such care.

Legislation as toothless and vague as R.M.P. could hardly have been expected to survive the harsh realities of local health politics.

The story of R.M.P. in New York City is a case study of what happens to such frail federal legislation in the hands of local medical barons. The elitist assumption that medical schools would take leadership in reorganizing medicine ignored the existing role conflicts among the medical empires. Some were too busy building their own private regional empires to bother with the regional service networks R.M.P. envisioned. Others were afraid to tarnish their academic research and educational excellence through involvement in regional schemes. The result, in New York, has been a disaster. There is almost nothing to show for the three million dollars that the medical schools spent for planning in the first two and a half years of the program. The record of the New York Metropolitan Regional Medical Program (N.Y.M.-R.M.P.) at a glance reveals:

(1) Only three projects have been approved and funded. One, the pediatric pulmonary center of Babies Hospital at Columbia, is a failure. The second, the Mobile Coronary Care Unit at another hospital, is a poorly conceived demonstration. The third, a course in modern techniques for cancer diagnosis and therapy at a specialized cancer hospital, is an expensive way of making available the education the hospital should have been providing all along.

(2) No plan or set of priorities has been established for the metropolitan region. What data has been collected on the needs of the region is meager and superficial.

(3) During the last part of 1968 and the first part of 1969,

almost all the central staff has left the program. The associate director was the first to go. He was soon followed by
the director, the director of program development, the
director of administration and organization, and finally by
the director of research and evaluation. When a new director was finally found for the $48,000-a-year post, the lapse
in leadership had already cost over $200,000 in grant exten-
sions just to keep N.Y.M.-R.M.P. nominally alive.

In New York City the attitude of the medical schools
doomed R.M.P. from the start. For openers, the deans of
the New York City medical schools met and decided that
they were not going to participate in the program. R.M.P.
did not really offer them much. There were no funds for
new construction, nor was there any opportunity to take
over and staff hospitals. Instead, they were supposed to
strengthen small community hospitals by cooperating
with them. In many cases, the hospitals that they were
supposed to aid were in competition with the medical
schools for staff, research money, and new facilities. Now
the medical schools were to associate not only with strong
hospitals but also with the weak hospitals and the lowest
level of practitioners—groups which they had systematically excluded in their drive to build centers of excellence.

Curiously enough, it was the elite, isolationist Cornell
Medical College which was one of the first medical schools
in the city to change its mind and apply to plan a Regional
Medical Program. Part of the reason was that Memorial
Hospital for Cancer, which is closely affiliated with Cornell, felt that it could get some money from R.M.P. for
some of its already existing programs. It looked to nearby
Cornell as the medical school with which to form a Regional Medical Program. Downstate Medical School also

applied to organize a Regional Medical Program at the urging of some of its affiliated hospitals. Subsequently several other medical schools, also began writing applications for their own R.M.P.

Washington, however, insisted that, in keeping with congressional intent, "there should not be a region for each medical school." This decision was made in part to avoid the fragmentation of a natural region, New York City, and in part to avoid the political problem of deciding how to parcel Manhattan among its five medical schools. So the medical schools and the New York Academy of Medicine formed a corporation, the Associated Medical Schools of Greater New York, Inc., which was awarded a two-year planning grant for the New York Metropolitan Regional Medical Program. Cornell Dean John Deitrick was chosen to be president for the first year of planning.

The deans, although not enthusiastic about the program, were determined to control it through their new corporation. Of the various agencies other than medical schools that expressed interest in becoming trustees of the corporation, only the prestigious New York Academy of Medicine had enough political clout to get a seat. The Health and Hospital Planning Council (see chapter XIV) and the City's Health Services Administration were relegated to the back seats. They were only given representation on the advisory committee, along with the medical societies.

Under the national R.M.P. guidelines, this advisory committee was supposed to be a broadly representative professional group with power to prevent the program from neglecting the interests of health care providers not allied with the medical schools. It was to have had the responsibility for approving all applications for operational grants. But the deans made it a subservient group. As a recent federal audit declared, the deans "were in a position to dictate the decisions and evaluations required of the advisory committee."

In 1968, seventeen members of the forty-five member advisory committee were connected to medical schools or to their affiliates. The remainder of the committee was hardly representative of the community. The so-called public representatives were mostly Wall Street business-men and philanthropists. Also listed as a public representa-tive was the vice-president of the Health and Hospital Planning Council. Medicine's own out-groups were ex-cluded from membership. There were no unaffiliated physicians on the committee and there were no repre-sentatives from the smaller voluntary hospitals or the pro-prietary (profit-making) hospitals. As if all these safeguards against unwelcome advice were not enough, the deans kept for themselves the powers of choosing a chairman for the advisory committee and changing its by-laws.

Having emasculated the advisory committee, the deans next turned to weakening the program's central staff, which, according to their own grant proposal, was sup-posed to be "responsible for coordinating the activities carried on by the staff located at the medical schools and for the proper allocation and reallocation of resources within the project." Instead, the deans set up a decentral-ized structure, resting heavily on staff located in the various medical schools. They gave their appointed central direc-tor no say in the selection of the local staff regional coor-dinators. One of the coordinators was not even seen by the director during the year he was there. The deans also decided that the coordinators were actually their repre-sentatives as well as staff of the project. So the coordinators often substituted for the deans at the meetings of the trustees. The director often found his "staff" acting as his boss.

One of the more important things decentralized under this administrative structure was the money. Each school (and the academy as well) raked off tens of thousands of dollars each year to pay for whatever local R.M.P. staff it wanted. The sums ranged from about $34,000 for Cornell to $100,000 for Downstate Medical Center. In addition, the schools padded their expenses with overhead charges, which have never been satisfactorily explained, to the federal R.M.P. buraucracy. For one medical center, these overhead charges amounted to almost as much as the R.M.P. staff salaries, an extra $34,000.

When the central staff did try to take initiative to broaden the interest of the program, their efforts were obstructed by the deans. For instance, the deans objected to the involvement of the central staff with the Model Cities Program. When the staff member who was the liaison between the programs left R.M.P., the involvement with Model Cities was quietly forgotten. The deans also frowned upon the attempts of the director to fund the Student Health Project in New York. Although the Student Health Project was finally funded by R.M.P., it was not funded by the metropolitan program, but by Washington directly.

When the central staff suggested to the deans that the medical schools become more involved in the continuing education of community physicians who had been barred from hospital application by the medical schools and voluntary hospitals, they met vigorous resistance and even resentment. John Deitrick, who was then president of the board of trustees, suggested that "the larger voluntary hospitals might undertake a program to upgrade medical education by providing better training for house and attending staffs and allied health personnel." The medical schools were thought not to have a role and the unaffiliated doctors were to be ignored.

In October of 1968 the director was finally fired for being too independent of the deans. Beginning with the appointment of a new director in March of 1969, the New York R.M.P. underwent a reorganization which, if it accomplished anything, strengthened the control of the medical schools. The advisory committee was made nominally more representative, not by changing its membership, but by increasing its size from forty-five to eighty-eight—with an eventual total of 120 in the offing. This change actually strengthened the medical schools' grip, since an advisory committee of nearly a hundred is essentially a rubber stamp. Real power remains in the executive committee, which is just as dominated by the medical schools as were the old advisory and executive committees. Just to make sure the newly expanded advisory group doesn't get out of hand, it's chaired by Dr. Frederick Eagle, dean of the New York Medical College and president of the Associated Medical Schools of Greater New York.

Although the medical schools fought for absolute control of R.M.P., they have provided no leadership to get the program moving. The deans declared that they were responsible for policy determination for R.M.P., that they would set the priorities, determine the program direction, and the philosophy of the local R.M.P. But they haven't. They had doubts about R.M.P. from the beginning and these doubts have not given way to enthusiasm. One dean is quoted as having said, "Sometimes when I go to bed at night, I hope that when I wake up in the morning, R.M.P. will have disappeared." As a result of the lack of leadership,

priorities were never established and very little planning
was done.

The annual report of New York R.M.P. suggests that
the medical schools spent what little energy they could
spare for R.M.P. dividing up the turf. Downstate Medical
Center got Brooklyn; Einstein, the Bronx; Columbia took
upper Manhattan; Mount Sinai and New York Medical
college shared East Harlem and part of Queens; Cornell
got Westchester and the rest of Queens. Actually, of
course, the medical schools did not develop boroughwide
or regional responsibilities just because of R.M.P. The
medical school R.M.P. coordinators, whose function was
supposedly to stimulate grant applications in poor institutions throughout their entire region, rarely bothered to
look outside their own institutions and affiliates. In New
York City, then, R.M.P. served only to strengthen the
existing medical empires.

Small hospitals, which are unaffiliated with medical
schools and which fall between the city's empires, have
been effectively shut out of R.M.P. When it comes to grant
writing, it's hard enough for a small hospital to compete
with a grant-padded major medical center. But it's virtually impossible to compete with major medical centers
which have special relations to R.M.P. staff and leadership.
R.M.P. staff were not very sympathetic to the requests of
small hospitals for more help in writing grants. In an
editorial in the R.M.P. newsletter, the R.M.P. director
wondered disdainfully: "If the applicants have neither the
time nor talent to describe clearly what will be done by the
project, will they have the ability to conduct it?" Once a
grant is written, it faces a volunteer review committee
composed largely of experts from the major teaching hospitals, who have tended to fund their own institutions. One

doctor was actually a member of the committee which reviewed his own grant application. A pulmonary center was awarded to Columbia rather than to a small hospital in Queens because of Columbia's "proven ability." Thus the rich get richer.

Considering the lack of leadership in the program, it is not surprising that only fifty-one project applications were received by New York R.M.P. from the local regions in the first two years. The overwhelming majority of these came from the seven medical schools, and one-half were from a single medical school, Downstate. Most of the proposals were for highly technical projects serving narrow medical subspecialties that were of interest only to the medical schools themselves. Few carried any hint of regionwide applicability, or even medical necessity. In fact, the deans themselves found only twelve projects which would not be embarrassing to send to federal R.M.P. for approval and possible funding. Only three have been funded at this writing. The three projects which have been funded after all this are little more than a mockery of both the planning process which is supposed to be part of R.M.P. and of the purpose of the entire program. One of these, the application for the Pediatric Pulmonary Center at Babies Hospital at Columbia, was quickly solicited and pushed through the advisory committee. It appears that central R.M.P. in Washington was given some money earmarked for pulmonary centers that had to be spent within a month. Washington asked the R.M.P. in New York to quickly dig up a pulmonary center. The other funded project, the Mobile Coronary Care Unit at St. Vincent's Hospital, was planned long before R.M.P. was established in New York. When the Heart Association didn't fund it, it was submitted to R.M.P.

In its application, Babies Hospital proposed a pediatric pulmonary center that appeared to be exactly the kind of integration and extension of services the R.M.P. was supposed to encourage. Babies proposed to extend the use of specialized procedures in the diagnosis and management of chronic respiratory diseases by fusing a number of existing clinics and laboratories into a single pediatric pulmonary disease center and tightening its existing affiliation arrangements with six metropolitan hospitals. However, a federal audit has shown that Babies Hospital has done little to implement its proposal. It took the money, hired a few more researchers and continued functioning as usual.

The Mobile Coronary Care Unit, a specially equipped ambulance at St. Vincent's, will probably never benefit anyone but the Greenwich Village community served by St. Vincent's. It provides on-the-spot emergency treatment to heart attack victims. An expensive and therefore hard-to-imitate demonstration project, it is basically a luxury. The money could have been better spent upgrading the training of ambulance attendants throughout the city or improving the existing inadequate arrangements among hospitals for the acceptance of ambulance patients.

The one other project in New York that is funded by R.M.P. is the Study of the Care of Cancer Patients at Memorial Hospital. This did not have to bother with advisory committee review and approval, however. Washington made funding the Memorial project, which was begun long before R.M.P. started, part of the original R.M.P. planning grant.

During the next few months, nine new project proposals were approved at the local level and sent in for national approval. Of these, four were disapproved on a federal level, three were approved but not funded (R.M.P. nationally began to run out of money just as New York R.M.P. finally got off the ground), two are still in the review cycle, and one has been conditionally approved. Those which are approved one way or another include: two projects for continuing education of health professionals in stroke and cancer, a "study of services and facilities for respiratory diseases in the New York metropolitan R.M.P. area," and a diffuse project to plan for the training of new kinds of health professionals. After two-and-a-half years and three million dollars, that was the best R.M.P. had to offer to New York City.

The story of New York Metropolitan R.M.P. differs only in details from the history of R.M.P. in the nation's fifty-five other R.M.P. regions. Everywhere, R.M.P.'s have taken on the characteristics of the region's local power structure. Regions with the largest concentration of medical schools, such as Chicago and New York, took the longest to get rolling, since all the inter-medical school rivalries had to be ironed out. In other, more rural regions where medical societies hold sway, R.M.P.s sprang up somewhat more rapidly, usually generating programs of benefit only to the local private doctors, despite the overwhelming need for coping with rural health problems. Without a single exception, local R.M.P.s have managed to exclude representatives of low-income or middle-income health care consumers from both their staffs and their advisory groups.

Everywhere, local medical power struggles and just plain foot-dragging occupied the first year or two of R.M.P.'s existence. It took until 1968 (two years after the R.M.P. bill was passed) just to get the full fifty-five regions into the organizational phase, and that amounted to little more than establishing a *modus vivendi* between contentious institutions and medical societies. So, swamped with money it could not spend, the federal R.M.P. bureaucracy embarked headlong on a policy of funding any project submitted for approval, with little regard to quality or relevance to any overall plan. About forty percent of total R.M.P. funds went for local R.M.P. staff and their expenses, and the rest went largely for continuing education programs for private physicians, coronary care units for small hospitals, tumor registries, and a host of gadgetry and services peripheral to any real modification of the delivery of health services. Nowhere was there any serious attempt to plan for regionally integrated patterns of health services, or even for "regional cooperative arrangements" —but then, R.M.P. offered no dollar incentives for planning.

R.M.P.s locally have made no progress towards the rationalizing or coordinating of medical services. In fact, in many cases R.M.P. has probably contributed to the existing fragmentation and irrationality. Examples abound of regions purchasing equipment through R.M.P. which they lack the technical expertise to use, or buying sophisticated electronic equipment for small hospitals which lack basic supplies and equipment for ordinary run-of-the-mill diseases. One hospital acquired expensive audio-visual equipment and facilities for film production, which completely duplicated the equipment already present in a nearby hospital. A southern R.M.P. region purchased a computer for a cancer registry and then was unable to find programmers to run it. The metropolitan District of Columbia region, whose city claims the worst health statistics in the country, proposed as one of its R.M.P. projects a twelve million-dollar expenditure to use the communications satellite for beaming advanced medical education programs to the entire world!

Unable to spend even the money that had been appropriated in its first two years of life, the R.M.P. budget was drastically reduced in fiscal year 1969. With the advent of Nixon's domestic austerity program, there seems to be no chance of future increases in R.M.P. funding. There is a saying in Washington: A level-funded program (i.e., one whose budget is not increased) is a dead program. For R.M.P., level-funding is probably a reliable portent of final doom. Without additional funds, it will be impossible for R.M.P. to hold the tenuous interest of the medical schools and research centers now involved. Never having emerged as a power structure on its own, and reflecting only the clash of already-existing powers, R.M.P. cannot hope to be saved by any organized pressure on the government. There is no R.M.P. lobby; there are few powerful friends. Confusion over allocation of health planning functions between R.M.P. and Comprehensive Health Planning further reduces the chance of survival. But then, anything worth surviving in R.M.P. died four years ago, in the drastic operation which transformed the De Bakey commission report into law. R.M.P., *R.I.P.*

XVI

THE EMPIRE HAS NO CLOTHES

The sixties took medicine out of the doctor's black bag and transformed it into a growth industry. Empires sprang up where before there had been only scattered fortresses, and engorged doctors, hospitals, health centers, and their dependent populations of human "material". Public spending on health grew from an irregular trickle into the geyser of Medicaid and Medicare, creating vast new areas of expansion for the empires and for the health products industry. The federal government brought forth potentially sweeping reorganizational programs to rationalize and harness the dynamism of this newer, bigger health system.

The empires, the medical-industrial complex, and the money which spawned them, are still big. But the "Health New Deal"—the mid-sixties' gesture towards a more rational and egalitarian health system—lies in wreckage across the land. Medicare is a disappointment; Medicaid is a scandal. Regional Medical Programs and Comprehensive Health Planning are two new overlays of irrationality on top of the system they were meant to restructure. Even the brave new federally financed neighborhood health and mental health centers have settled down as imperial fiefdoms or closed up shop on account of community problems.

Consumers, even the ones who don't read the glowing descriptions of the health industry in *The Wall Street Journal*, are aware that there's a new bigness to the health system: the bills are bigger; and the lines of people waiting for care are longer. The consumer's over-all impression is one of increased scarcity, not of growth. The proportion of general practitioners to the total population falls year after year, with no help in sight from any new kinds of supplementary medical personnel. Medical responsibility to the patient as a whole person declines with the emergence of each new hair-splitting medical subspecialty. There are more and more life-giving or beautifying drugs and devices to consume, but there is less and less chance of assessing their worth, or paying the price.

1970, like 1965, is bringing more and more talk of restructuring the health system. So far, the strategy advanced by the medical insiders and concerned outside interests seems to consist of redoubling the mistakes of the past: Medicaid, Medicare and Blue Cross taught that open-handed public subsidy of an unregulated health system is not only wasteful in the short-run, but leaves permanent distortions on the pattern of health services delivery. So the medical "reformers" plan to consolidate Medicaid, Medicare and all other insurance schemes into one giant package, to sanction it with public authority, and to dignify it with the name "National Health Insurance." Empires have proved their inability to deliver, whether the task is something as limited as operating a community hospital or health center or as open-ended as creating a regional medical program. So the medical reformers propose that a "rational" health system is one in which *all* the nation's health services would be arranged into imperial domains, or regional health authorities, under the trusteeship of medical schools and major teaching hospitals. The philosophy guiding the medical reform effort is like the philosophy guiding the American effort in Vietnam: if something was a mistake in the past, it deserves another try, but on a much bigger scale.

Not everyone is ready to go along with this. Just as the American soldier in Vietnam doesn't care whether he is participating in something called pacification, Vietnamization, or annihilation, the factory worker doesn't care whether the money taken out of his paycheck for health goes to something called Blue Cross, Metropolitan Life Insurance Company, or National Health Insurance. And the big city clinic-user couldn't care less that his neighborhood hospital is part of an integrated, modern, medical empire. In fact, more and more people, veterans of Medicaid and Medicare, are not even interested in seeing new money appropriated for health. It's harder and harder to find a place to spend it, and sometimes it doesn't even seem to be worth the trouble of trying.

What's come over people is not, as one New York medical emperor claimed, "the traditional public apathy about health," but a new understanding of the depth of the changes necessary to create a humane and effective health system. Brilliant new technical fixes, no matter how well-promoted, just don't sell anymore. Fewer and fewer people really believe that new arrangements like national health insurance, prepaid group practices, or regionalization, will be the wonder drugs which will save the health system. Like heart transplants, all these miraculous new techniques for rationalizing and vitalizing the system have begun to look like last-ditch efforts to advertise a failing system to a jaded public. No one is interested in reshufflings and repackagings of the same old fragments. No one is interested in renovating a building which ought to be condemned.

The alternatives are just barely beginning to be heard. They do not have the appeal of technological gimmickry, or the dignity conferred by powerful and respected spokesmen, but they are simple: according to a growing movement of health workers, students and consumers, meaningful change must begin with a reordering of the priorities of the health system. Patient care must be put first; otherwise no amount of new reform—stable financing, new manpower, more efficient patterns of delivery of care—can mean anyting to the patient. Research and training are important, but they must be financed and organized so that they are not parasitical on the care of the poor. Profits must be phased out, for they have no place in an enterprise in which human life is at stake. A publicly accountable system must replace private enterprise in providing all health care and health products. When the priorities of the health system have been reversed, then it will make sense to discuss the niceties of hospital planning, or clinic administration, or group practice design.

More and more consumers are beginning to think that this approach makes sense. The only trouble is that they haven't found anyone willing to do it for them. Traditionally, health care is something that the public entrusts to hospital trustees, scientists, medical school deans, drug company executives, government health officials, and the like, and none of these is about to sacrifice profits, prestige, or personal empire in the cause of public service. The movement which is demanding change has begun to understand that only it can provide the leadership for change. The obstacles are almost paralyzingly huge—the almost impenetrable technological mystique of health care and health professionals, the increasing consolidation and monopolization of the health industry, and the political authority of the imperial and industrial trustees of the health system. But what is at stake is worth the struggle and the new responsibility.

The movement for revolutionary restructuring of the health system is in direct continuity with the larger American movement for a more democratic, egalitarian society. One stream comes out of the medical and nursing schools, which, starting in the late sixties, began to see students who bore no resemblance to the straight-laced, conservative classes of previous decades. The late-sixties' student entered professional school in the wake of four years' exposure of campus Vietnam, civil rights, and student power protests. By 1968, the student movement was busy "bringing the war home," to issues of university complicity in imperialism and racism; campus R.O.T.C. programs, limited admissions for blacks, university defense research, etc. A sizeable minority of the new crop of medical and nursing students started out with the suspicion that their professional schools were no more likely than the university to be innocent of racist and imperialist functions. At the same time, a new majority of medical and nursing students—certainly not radicals—came with idealistic expectations of learning how to serve, not how to make money or do research or be bureaucrats. The medical and nursing schools did the rest—thwarting the expectations of the liberals and confirming the suspicions of the radicals. The medical student movement became large enough to support its own national organization, the Student Health Organization. Other medical and nursing students, along with recently graduated health professionals, poured into the Medical Committee for Human Rights. By 1970 the

growing movement is large enough to support several publications around the country and has been strong enough
to carry off militant actions around health issues in a number of cities.

A newer but fast-growing element of the health movement is the women's liberation movement. Starting in the
mid-sixties, more and more young women, veterans of
peace and civil rights activities, began to look into their
own oppression as women in a male-dominated society.
For a year or so the movement was barely visible, as it
busied itself with one-to-one organizing around the issues
of women's sexual exploitation in the home, the workplace
and in the media. In 1968, the movement surfaced with
organized attacks on the institutional sources of male domination, such as women's magazines and cosmetics companies. Women's groups in Boston, New York, and
Washington took on the health system as a prime target.
As health workers, women occupy subservient and under-
paid slots: seventy percent of the nation's health workers
are women, but only seven percent of the nation's physicians are women. As health consumers, women use more
medical care than men (mainly because of childbirth and
childrearing) and are subjected to specifically "sexist" (the
analog of "racist") indignities in the course of getting that
care. Women's liberation groups are increasingly taking
action around specifically femininist demands—dignified
obstetrical and gynecological care and legal abortions, for
example—as well as more general demands for low-cost,
high quality health care.

The medical students' and the women's branches of the
health movement are largely white. But by far the largest
element of the health movement is black and brown, including both health workers and health consumers. Blacks,

Puerto Ricans and Mexican-Americans have always been at the very bottom of the health system—exploited as workers to support the hospitals financially, and exploited as patients to support hospitals' research and teaching activities. The idea of doing anything about it goes back to the civil rights sit-ins in the early sixties. The energy of the civil rights movement quickly spilled over into other areas: demands on schools for the right to education, demands on welfare agencies for the right to an adequate income, and, more recently, demands on health institutions for the newly perceived right to health care. In the mid-sixties, as the civil rights movement grew into the black liberation movement, the demands began to shift from equal rights in a white-run society to all-out self-determination for black communities. The demands put on health institutions were no longer just for more and better services, but for community participation in the planning and priority-setting of health centers, hospitals and even medical schools. As of 1970, New York had more than a dozen black and Puerto Rican neighborhood organizations concerned solely with health. Even in smaller cities, like Fresno and El Paso, and in Southern rural areas, there are the beginnings of black and brown movements for community control of local health institutions.

The message of civil rights movement was not lost on black health workers either. Starting in the early and mid-sixties, unions such as New York's Local 1199, Drug and Hospital Workers, and the American Federation of State, County, and Municipal Employees, began a massive hospital organizing drive, borrowing the techniques and even the personnel of the larger civil rights movement. People like the Southern Christian Leadership Conference's Reverend Ralph Abernathy and Coretta Scott King (Mrs.

Martin Luther King, Jr.) joined in the organizing drives,
linking the issues of civil rights and the right to a decent
living. Despite these promising associations, the unions
representing hospital workers—from the Teamsters to 1199
—have shown little interest in health issues beyond the
bread-and-butter concerns of their membership. But this in
itself has been an important contribution. Workers who
make a decent living and have some degree of job security
have at least the possibility of struggling for career advancement or for better community health programs. In
New York, where some two-thirds of the hospital workers
are union members, workers in a number of institutions
have joined with community groups in demands for better
services and greater community involvement. In other
health institutions, workers have formed black caucuses or
radical caucuses to struggle for better services and greater
democracy within their health facilities.

Only in the last couple of years have these separate
streams—the medical and nursing students', women's, and
black and brown communities' and workers' movements
—begun to come together as a single health movement.
White, middle-class, medical students realized that they
would be imitating the patronizing style of their medical
school mentors if they worked for, rather than with, the
low-income community served by the medical school-hospital complex. Students in New York University, Columbia, and Einstein Medical Schools in New York, have
gone off-campus to find leadership from neighborhood
health organizations. In some cases, neighborhood consumer groups have sought out the radical medical students,
and enlisted them in community struggles. Women's
groups have joined forces with black women consumers,
as in Washington, D.C., or linked up with black women

hospital workers, as in Chicago. Health workers' groups are making contact with medical students and young doctors' organizations within the same institution, and with community groups outside.

What is emerging is a sense of common struggle, and the outlines of a common program. Health workers, including medical students, and health consumers obviously have different and even potentially conflicting interests. The basis for consensus is that health workers cannot really do their job, if their job is health care, in a system structured around profits, research, and education. At the same time health consumers cannot get good care, on a dignified basis, from a system that is internally hierarchical and oppressive to its workers. The kind of joint program which has been taking shape in New York and other cities calls for reorganizing and redirecting of the health system: health care should be free at the point of delivery (i.e., the costs should be borne by the entire society, through the tax system). Hospitals should move beyond their present "first aid" emphasis and focus on preventive health services. Internally, health institutions should be run democratically, with decision-making shared by health professionals, nonprofessionals and community people. Outside forces, such as trustees and philanthropic organizations, should be deposed, since they contribute little to the health service process (not even money any more). Doctors should be salaried employees, not free entrepreneurs. Medical schools and other schools of health services should open their doors to all black, brown, and white women applicants and white working-class youths, and should provide opportunities for professional training, up to the M.D. level, for all interested health workers—nurses to orderlies. In short, the health system should be recreated as a democratic enterprise, in which patients are participants (not customers or objects) and health workers, from physicians to aides, are all colleagues in a common undertaking.

An ambitious program for a movement which is still so young and small? Maybe, but the chances are that both the movement and its program will grow explosively in the next few years. Medical students, young women, and blacks as a whole are not the only groups that are oppressed by the American health system. More and more ordinary, white, middle-class Americans are finding themselves up against a health system which promises far more than it delivers, and costs far more than it is worth. The first stirrings of discontent have been heard, and noted, by unions, management and government, but the chances of a meaningful response from them are slight. As the health system gets bigger, more industrialized, and more centralized, the differences between poor and middle-class, or black and white consumers begin to blur. No one is making it, and everyone has a stake in the creation of a revolutionary, people-oriented health system.

XVII

THE STUDENT HEALTH ORGANIZATION: BRINGING IT ALL BACK HOME

The Student Health Organization Projects . . . represent some of the most innovative and inspiring chapters in the history of America's healing arts in reaching out to the poor. I would like to see your good work multiplied manyfold.

Hubert H. Humphrey, Vice-President of the United States, February 1968.

We have certainly seen enough evidence that the members of the Student Health Organization should have been the last persons in the world to receive taxpayers' money [for their projects].

Roman Pucinski, Illinois congressman, December 1969.

It took less than two years for the establishment to change its mind about the Student Health Organization. In those two years, the Student Health Organization changed from a Peace Corps-style community service project into a radical political organization.

The Student Health Organization (S.H.O.) was founded in 1965 by some sixty-five students from twenty-five schools of medicine, nursing, dentistry, and social work. It was the product of reaction: reaction to the passive and pecuniary orientation of the majority of health science students; reaction to the vacuity of existing student health professional organizations, such as the Student American Medical Association;* reaction to the authoritarian and sterile education offered by professional schools. The problem, as S.H.O.'s founders saw it, was that medical education systematically recreates the hierarchy of medical practice—separating medical students from students in allied professions, and separating all health students from the patient community they are supposedly learning to serve. But, instead of attacking the problem at its source—the medical schools themselves—the early S.H.O. members looked for ways out of the restrictive atmosphere of medical school. Following the lead of the civil rights movement,

---

*S.A.M.A., the Student American Medical Association, was founded under A.M.A. auspices in 1950. When S.H.O. was founded in 1965, S.A.M.A. did little more than offer medical students life insurance and discounts on new car purchases. Under challenge from S.H.O., S.A.M.A. has developed a new liberal facade. But S.A.M.A. still excludes nursing, dental, and social work students; it still receives close to $230,000 a year from advertising from drug companies in its magazine. It continues to claim membership of a vast majority of medical students, although most schools do not give the student a choice about joining S.A.M.A., but simply deduct S.A.M.A. dues from his tuition. S.A.M.A. officers brag that they have developed a "multi-million dollar conglomerate" by garnering money from private and governmental grants, over and above their drug advertising haul. Yet their community service projects fail and their membership is not moved by community experience. (S.A.M.A.'s president said: "This government-sponsored volunteer program was sold to us on the theory that if we saw Appalachia we would come back and serve it. That's too simplistic. Appalachia is not a viable option for medical students wanting to get ahead.") S.A.M.A. may have declared independence from its parent organization, but it shares the congenital defects bequeathed by the A.M.A.—narrow professionalism and an all-consuming profit motive.

they turned to the urban ghetto and the migrant labor camp as settings where students could relate to patients and to each other more effectively and democratically.

A few months after its founding, S.H.O. swung into action with its first summer service program, financed by a sizeable federal grant. Over ninety medical, nursing, dental, and social work students gathered in California to study and serve the poor of the state. In Watts, students conducted an audio-visual screening program for 4,000 children in the Headstart program. In the San Joaquin Valley, students acted as patient advocates for migrant workers, bringing people to hospital clinics and demanding that they be seen without interminable waiting. Working with state and county health departments, students designed and executed surveys which exposed the poor health of ghetto residents. The student participants ended the summer more enthusiastic than they had begun; the gaps between student and community, student and patient, and medical student and nursing student, seemed to be closing. The next year, 1967, 260 health science students worked in three student health projects, in California, Chicago, and New York City. By 1968, projects had proliferated to nine cities with over 600 student participants.

There was a lot of variation among the summer projects, but they all, one way or another, achieved what they had set out to do. Students got a first-hand exposure to the health problems of the poor and a glimpse of what the health system looks like from the bottom up. Medical, nursing, and other students learned to work together as teams—although these teams were usually dominated by the medical students. But there were some unexpected irritations. Summer projects were expensive, requiring a total of over one million dollars in 1968. Since the projects were largely student-administered, S.H.O. leaders had to spend days writing funding proposals and traveling around the country trying to sell them to foundations and government agencies. Then, since projects relied so heavily on government funding, especially from the Office of Economic Opportunity, they smacked of the antipoverty program—an association which, the students learned, was not always helpful in poverty areas.

Irritated by the administrative form of the projects, S.H.O. members gradually began to question the projects' basic function as well. Some students began to point out that the projects served the medical schools and the government perhaps even more effectively than they served the poor. Medical schools found that the summer projects were a cheap and effortless way to improve their image in neighboring ghettos—certainly a lot easier than giving better care at the medical school's affiliated hospitals. Likewise, the government found it a lot cheaper to fund an S.H.O. summer project than to build and staff a health center for an urban ghetto. As a further benefit, the projects played a useful role gathering information about community power structures which would not otherwise be available to government agencies.

Stanford students were the first to cut out from government funding and medical school affiliations. In a spring 1968 open letter announcing their decision to carry on a small independent project on their own, Stanford S.H.O. wrote:

> We are developing an increasingly large base of medical people who are understanding that the problems of community health are political problems, problems of power and control over the institutions which affect one's day to day life; that

they are not simply the problems of applying new technologies to backward areas. . . . If, as individuals, we understand and believe in the movements for self determination and local control in poor communities, we must be careful not to work through organizations or projects which are constructed antithetically to these notions; the structure of an institution may make its overall effect oppressive and authoritarian even though its members try to act otherwise. Ironically, just as S.H.O. members are becoming aware of this danger, the structure of the organization and the forms of the projects are developing in the opposite direction. While on the individual level, we are placing increasing emphasis on close relations with community groups . . . the overall structure, policy, and direction of our projects is being determined by a coalition of students, university and the federal government.

The next clash occurred in New York, where students at Einstein College of Medicine demanded that the medical school surrender its policy-setting control over the summer project. Just before the 1968 project was to get off the ground, its student directors demanded that a board consisting of students, community residents and medical school faculty, each with equal vote, be set up to guide the project. But Dr. Martin Cherkasky, chairman of the Community Medicine Department at Albert Einstein College of Medicine and nominal recipient of the government grant for the student project, insisted that he maintain a veto over all activities of the summer project. Undercut in their efforts to create a small island of community participation and control within the medical empire, the student directors resigned. To go ahead with the project, they announced, would have been to serve as a public relations front for the medical school in the community. All over the country S.H.O. students were coming to the same conclusion: S.H.O. summer projects were the creatures of the medical school establishment.

S.H.O. chapters in nine medical schools went ahead with summer projects in 1968 anyway, but the final disillusionment was not long in coming. Regional Medical Programs (see chapter XV), a major federal financier of the projects, called a meeting of the student directors from the nine projects to discuss ways of evaluating the summer projects. One of the prime evaluative mechanisms pushed by R.M.P. was that the students submit reports on their contacts with community organizations and community leaders. What better way to measure S.H.O.'s rapport with the communities it served, while, at the same time, helping R.M.P. identify community organizations for future grants? Nevertheless, some of the students saw the counterinsurgency potential of this request. How could they be sure that the information would not be used against, rather than for, the community groups and leaders they reported on? Some of the project directors acquiesced to R.M.P.'s request, but most developed their own evaluative schemes. All had been alerted to the government's stake in their projects.

The disenchantment which had been mounting for four years all came to a head at the 1968 S.H.O. National Assembly. More and more students criticized S.H.O. for involving itself only in summer projects, and criticized the summer projects themselves for being nothing more than "shitwork for the establishment." It was clear that the best S.H.O. leadership was tied up all year round raising money for the projects and spent the summer hassling about pay checks, bookkeeping and other administrative matters. For what purpose? To provide screening services that should be a part of the public health department or the medical school clinics? To survey the community and its health problems for the government and the university? To divert student discontent and activism from its source, within the medical and the nursing school, to the community? There was a growing realization that a coalition had unwittingly been formed between health science students, the university and the federal government; and that that coalition operated, as some students put it, "to make the community safe for the medical school."

As criticism of the summer student health projects increased, so too did the understanding that a large part of the health problems of the poor were caused by the very medical centers and schools in which students obtained their training. In urban ghetto areas, the medical school and its affiliated hospitals are often the only source of medical care. But medical schools have shown no signs of rising to meet this responsibility. In fact, as students at Columbia pointed out in 1969 leaflets "There is an institutionalized double standard of care at the Medical Center." Even at medical centers far more service-oriented than Columbia, students quickly learn about the two-class system of care: paying patients receive private care with all the amenities; poor patients are used, impersonally, for research and training. Since they are the beneficiaries of the training made possible by poor patients, medical students, no less than their schools, are agents of exploitation. One Philadelphia S.H.O. member gave up his medical education, announcing in a mimeographed statement

> I've had my fill of putting it to blacks. I learned to draw blood on old black ladies. I learned to do pelvics on young black women. I learned to do histories and physicals on black bodies and on a few wrinkled and run-down white ones. Now, in order to learn something about primary care, about long-term

outpatient care, I am faced again with waiting black faces in the hospital clinics. I am forced to participate in a system providing fragmented, second-rate care in the present, while loudly proclaiming the best possible care for future patients (mostly white, suburban folk, of course—that is, if you don't end up having no patients at all, as in research, public health or administration).

Most S.H.O. students, however, decided to stay in school and fight it out. Nationwide, S.H.O.'s thrust shifted from studying the community to studying the medical schools themselves. Medical schools' failure to provide (in their affiliated hospitals) high-quality care for the poor was easy enough to document. In addition, students began to recognize the role of medical school admissions policies in limiting the supply, and skewing the distribution, of physicians. Students in Boston pointed out in a 1968 pamphlet entitled "Crisis":

> 34 percent of all medical students come from families with income in the top 3 percent of the population; and only 2.2 percent of all medical students are black or brown. Only an economic and racial bias within admissions policies could account for these statistics.

Looking further for the forces which shaped the medical schools' service and admissions policies, S.H.O. chapters discovered a power structure far more intricate—and powerful—than anything they had encountered in poor communities: medical school and affiliated hospital boards of trustees are dominated by bankers, businessmen, insurance, and real estate executives, and drug and hospital supply company executives.

The more S.H.O. members learned about their medical schools, the more bankrupt the summer health projects looked. It was no longer possible to think of working in a coalition with the medical school and the government to serve the community. In fact, students began to think that the best way to serve the community was to stay where they were and change the medical schools. Summer service projects began to change into fall action projects. In Philadelphia, the students who had run the 1968 summer project launched a fall project to demand increased black admissions to the Philadelphia medical schools. Constituting themselves as the Committee on Black Admissions (C.B.A.), they demanded that one-third of the students admitted to the class of 1969 be blacks. When the medical school deans and trustees flatly refused to meet with the C.B.A., the students went out and found support among black community organizations and sympathetic professional groups. The coalition around C.B.A. formed their own admissions committee to interview black applicants and pressure the medical schools for their admission.

Although the medical schools never accepted the demand for one-third blacks, they were compelled to increase black enrollment, and in September, 1969, over five percent of the entering classes in Philadelphia medical schools were black. The battle of admissions was carried one step further in Boston, where in fall 1969, students articulated a demand for open admissions to all Boston area medical and nursing schools, for all minority group applicants from Massachusetts.

Students did not stop at admission policies. They began to challenge their medical centers' dual system of health care. At Columbia University's medical school, for instance, students took the initiative to pull together a joint student-community assault on Presbyterian Hospital (the teaching hospital affiliated with Columbia's medical school). One morning in the spring of 1969, twenty-five medical students, mostly S.H.O. members, took the very unprofessional step of walking into the waiting room of Presbyterian's outpatient clinic and passing out leaflets to the waiting patients. The leaflets listed some of the gross inadequacies of the clinic and urged patients to sign a petition and meet with the students to discuss what could be done. Over thirty patients signed up in the half-hour before the hospital security force arrived on the scene and forced the students out into the street. In the months that followed, the students held a series of meetings with patients and representatives of community organizations and decided to aim for a community-wide rally on the Presbyterian issue. The rally, held in the winter of 1969, brought out over four hundred community people, and resulted in the formation of a permanent health council to challenge Columbia-Presbyterian's priorities.

Medical services offered at affiliated hospitals are only one of the issues over which medical schools have come into conflict with their neighboring communities. In addition to their academic pursuits, most major medical schools, such as Columbia and Harvard, are real estate empires, steadily expanding into surrounding neighborhoods. Harvard Medical School began buying up nearby property for a new hospital complex in 1961. As a landlord, the medical school permitted housing conditions to deteriorate for eight years with the hope that residents would move out. In the spring of 1969, the Ad Hoc Committee of Harvard Students uncovered Harvard's long-term plan for expansion and published a detailed expose:

> We have been trying to show that the Affiliated Hospital Complex project [the new complex planned by Harvard] is

not formulated in the interests of the people living on the land
in which it is to be built; and that the priorities on which it is
based do not serve the interests of the low-income community
in which the center will lie. These deficiencies of the plan . . .
are not mere mistakes but the logical outgrowths of the economic system and power relationships of our society. The
centralized medical facility plan . . . is more oriented towards
the needs of relatively affluent patients than a decentralized
community health facility would be. This priority reflects the
fact that resources for medical facilities are administered in
large measure by privately supported and controlled corporations, which are responsive to the needs of their affluent sponsors and to the narrow professionalism of their staffs.
Furthermore, the poor lack the political power required to
bring about public allocation of adequate resources for their
medical care.

As a result of the student agitation, a community group
formed to defend the neighborhood, and Harvard's construction has not gotten off the drawing board.

The actions at Harvard, Columbia, and in Philadelphia
are a long way from the old S.H.O. summer projects.
Everywhere the story is the same: S.H.O. members are no
longer interested in serving as junior professionals, mis-
sionaries to the poor. They see their responsibility for community health going far beyond narrowly medical
problems, and the possibilities of action going far beyond
the provision of medical services. The old coalition of
health students, universities, and the federal government
has given way to a new coalition of students and community activists. And the motto has changed. Students are
now working "to make the medical school safe for the
community."

XVIII

THE HEALTH WORKERS REVOLT:

LINCOLN BRIGADE II

On the morning of March 5, 1969, more than 150 mental
health workers, led by black and Puerto Rican nonprofessionals, seized control of the Lincoln Hospital Mental
Health Services (L.H.M.H.S.) in New York. Nonprofessional workers replaced professionals in adminstrative ca-
pacities and as heads of services. While not all professionals
were enthusiastic about this role reversal, at least three
psychiatrists who were chiefs of services continued to
work as technical consultants to the dissident nonprofessionals for the entire two weeks of the occupation. Altogether, more than eighty percent of the staff, including
many professionals, participated in one or another phase of
the takeover and the occupation of mental health center.
In its proportions, the takeover had the character of a
popular uprising rather than a coup, but it occurred
smoothly and quietly, with only minor initial disruption of
patient services.

Dr. Harris B. Peck, director and designer of
L.H.M.H.S., and his two associate directors were the immediate targets of the workers' frustration. Ironically, only
days before the administrators were shut out of their
offices, an article by Dr. Peck had appeared in *Reader's*

Digest saying: "When there's a foot planted in the seat of my trousers to kick me out of here, I'll know we've succeeded. It will mean that the people want to take over the running of their own community. And that's the way it should be." After the takeover, however, Dr. Peck backtracked, declaring that while he still favored the principle of community control, "It's a long-term goal. We don't think it is possible to implement it at this time."

The entire national mental health establishment was caught off guard. The Lincoln Hospital Mental Health Services, an inner-city, community-based mental health center in New York's south Bronx was perhaps the most widely known institution of its kind in the nation. The project had been designated by the National Institute of Mental Health as one of eight national model mental health centers and lauded for its efforts to hire and train local people for "new careers" in mental health. Just the year before the takeover, the American Psychiatric Association honored the project with its silver achievement award.

The shock was severe. Health workers had applied the tactics of campus militants. Never before had health workers rebelled in the name of community control. And everything about the Lincoln mental health center had seemed guaranteed to safeguard it from confrontations. In its service programs and organizational structure, it was an innovative, community-oriented program. Its special program for hiring and training local people seemed so certain to win worker loyalty that the rebels later called it a pacification program. If this could happen at Lincoln Hospital Mental Health Services, then how about Lincoln Hospital itself? How safe were Einstein Medical College and Montefiore Medical Center, the centers of the empire of which the Lincoln mental health center was only one tiny outpost?

Lincoln Hospital is wedged into a rapidly decaying ghetto community. More than a third of a million people lived in the surrounding neighborhood of factories, congested traffic, and aging apartment houses. A large segment of the population is Puerto Rican, a smaller number is black, and a decreasing number is aging white. The rate of unemployment in this south Bronx neighborhood is double that of the borough as a whole. Only the most acute health problems reach the hospital—a hospital which is the most physically deteriorated, ill-equipped and understaffed of all the sparsely endowed New York municipal hospitals. Its totally inadequate emergency room—the second-busiest in the nation and the family doctor for many in the south Bronx—has helped earn Lincoln its reputation in the community as "the butchershop." Mental health services for Lincoln Hospital, which is affiliated with Albert Einstein College of Medicine (see chapters V and VI) were organized in 1963. The mental health services were first housed only in the hospital complex then expanded with funds from the Office of Economic Opportunity in the mid-sixties to include three storefront service centers.

The 140 nonprofessional L.H.M.H.S. workers, mostly black and Puerto Rican natives of the south Bronx were recruited and trained for novel new careers in mental health programs. Under the "new careers" program, underemployed or unemployed people were recruited with the promise of educational opportunities which would propel them up a career ladder and might even culminate in their becoming professional health workers. In fact, the first few years at L.H.M.H.S. showed that the health hierarchy was not ready to open its doors to the indigenous mob. The nonprofessionals were increasingly frustrated by the discrepancy between promises and hard realities. Although more than thirty Lincoln nonprofessionals received some kind of formal schooling, it was not only unrelated to their jobs, but very few received pay increments or job mobility which was commensurate with their academic advancement.

In the early days of the Lincoln mental health center, however, the workers' disappointment with the rungless career ladders was partially made up for by the feeling that they were doing socially meaningful work. Under professional supervision, the black and Puerto Rican nonprofessionals worked in the storefront units, which were often the staging ground for such innovative (and effective) mental health programs as voter registration drives and rent strikes. Under the direction of Einstein College of Medicine, however, the storefronts, publicly billed as community service centers, were primarily research-oriented. The L.H.M.H.S. rhetoric proudly proclaimed neighborhood centers stocked with nonprofessional mental health workers who could identify with the ghetto clients. But the nonprofessionals were more often required to extract extensive research data—often irrelevant to the client's problem—from the anxious residents who came in search of help. Only when the research aspect of the job was complete, was the nonprofessional free to use whatever time or energy he had left to deal with the patient's shoddy housing or missing welfare check. Despite all the handicaps, the nonprofessional storefront-based mental health workers did get out into the community to organize social actions. But in 1967, the O.E.O. grant was replaced with a National Institute of Mental Health grant, and the original social action emphasis shifted to a more conventional medical-psychiatric approach. In 1968 the storefront service centers were phased out. Though three neighborhood mental health clinics were promised and paid for by the new federal grant, only one had materialized by 1969, and the majority of the mental health services were meted out by a hospital-based clinic. Feelings not only of frustration and insecurity, but of betrayal as well added kindling to the workers' growing resentment.

As nonprofessional community mental health workers were moved from the storefronts back to the hospital, they began to raise questions not only about what was happening to all the grant money that was flowing through L.H.M.H.S., but about the relevance of any hospital-based service at all. One new careerist describes his frustration as follows.

> When I first came here we dealt with people's needs. If a man was depressed and he lived in a rat hole, we went out and we helped move him. We carried his bed on our backs. In other cases, we started putting pressure on landlords. And then the word came down from the 'man'. . . . We don't move patients anymore—Einstein says we're not covered by insurance. Pressure on landlords? We've been ordered to cool it. In the case of one of the landlords, word came from high up. We found out later that the landlord was a big contributor to Yeshiva." [Einstein College of Medicine is a branch of Yeshiva University.]

In May 1968, the nonprofessional workers staged a sit-in in the administrative offices of L.H.M.H.S. their demands ranged from instituting upgrading and educational programs to the ultimate demand that Dr. Peck follow up on a promise to gradually shift control of the mental health center from his office (and Einstein) to the Lincoln workers and the community. A few days later, service chiefs

and project heads demanded greater delegation of authority and more participation in policy-making for
L.H.M.H.S. The lower level professional staff followed up
with a work stoppage over cutbacks in salary increments.
Dr. Peck maintained that the community wasn't ready to
participate in governing the center. But he conceded that
there could be more internal democracy, promising staff
elections to a new "policy planning and review board."

The workers met all through the summer to hammer
out procedures and principles for the new board which
was to represent the interests of both professionals and
nonprofessionals as well as heads of service and administrators. The final plan was accepted by the entire staff including Dr. Peck. But on October 4, 1968, just one day before
the balloting, the general counsel of Yeshiva University
intervened to declare that the establishment of a staff
policy planning and review board involved a proposed
delegation of powers of the University and the College of
Medicine without authority of either the University's
Board of Trustees or the College's Board of Overseers, that
this authority could not be delegated beyond present limits
without their consent, and that the consent had not been
given.

The decisive language of this proclamation left little
doubt in the workers' minds that there would be no further
review. In the five months following, other complaints
accumulated. The grievances that loomed above all others
were those charging discrimination—against nonwhite
workers, and hence against the community. For one example, fewer than twenty-three of the total of 120 professionals on the staff were black or Puerto Rican. When a slot
opened up in 1968 for a social worker, four blacks applied
for the position. They were refused as not suitable because

of lack of experience, but, the dissidents claimed, a white social worker with little experience was hired. Subsequently, all of the four "unqualified" blacks who were turned down by L.H.M.H.S. were hired elsewhere to fill equivalent or higher positions than the proffered L.H.M.H.S. post. Another example of alleged L.H.M.H.S. racism grew out of the hard and fast rule that the job of community organizer must be filled by a college graduate. The rule, Lincoln workers say, was followed stringently when the applicants were black or Puerto Rican. However, when a middle-aged white union organizer applied for the position he was hired despite the fact that he had no degree.

The immediate trigger for the March 1969, takeover was the dismissal of four black, nonprofessional workers in unrelated disciplinary actions by the administration. Theoretically, it was the responsibility of the union, Local 1199 of Drug and Hospital Workers' Union, to protect the fired workers, but the union and the L.H.M.H.S. workers had a long history of mutual distrust. Back in the spring of 1968, when the workers first demanded a role in policy-making, 1199 had made no move to back the workers; in fact, the union organizers did their best to cool things. As a result, the workers felt they couldn't rely on the union, especially in a struggle which went beyond the usual bread-and-butter issues. All that was left was to take matters into their own hands and directly confront the administration with their grievances.

The workers were impelled to action out of their own frustrations and disappointments with the mental health center—its gross misuse of funds, its rigid internal hierarchy, and its unresponsiveness to the community, which was also the home of many of the nonprofessional workers.

They chose the tactic of an occupation and work-in rather than a wildcat strike to show the community that they were concerned about improved services and not merely about increased pay or other economic demands. Once they had seized power in the health center the workers made immediate efforts to enlist the community—from established leaders to patients and their families—to share control of the "community" mental health center. For the month that the workers' revolt lasted, the Lincoln mental health center was the only thing approaching community-worker control of a major service institution in the nation.

The dissident workers—a coalition of nonprofessionals and professionals—made some eleven demands, among which were that the four workers who had been fired be reinstated with pay, and that the original intent of the new careers program be fulfilled by instituting a general upgrading program for all nonprofessionals. But the demands which were to become central were the call for the removal of L.H.M.H.S.'s director, Dr. Peck and his associate directors, the demand for the establishment of the policy planning and review board, and the call for "a meaningful community board with significant decision-making power and responsibilities over the administration and policies of Lincoln Hospital and L.H.M.H.S."

The workers set up a command post in the administrative offices. During the first few days, they were inundated with news reporters, volunteers, and curious community people. Despite the furor, the services continued to function. But three days after the occupation, the city Department of Hospitals and the Community Mental Health Board declared the services closed, saying that the ousted Einstein administrators could not be held medically responsible for the services. The workers refused to leave their posts, and, within a few hours a directive arrived from Einstein, warning the professionals among the occupiers that they would be subject to malpractice suits if they continued to work in an unauthorized medical facility. The threat was far-fetched—even some of the city health officials felt that it was unusually vindictive—but it put a scare into the professionals and split many of them from the other workers. The remaining dissident professionals withdrew from the mental health clinic in the hospital's main building and joined the nonprofessionals in setting up services in an annex building. The annex and the one neighborhood mental health clinic continued to offer skeletal services and were to be the worker strongholds for the next two weeks.

On Monday, March 17, the city learned that state and federal funds were jeopardized by the closing, and ordered the hospital-based services to reopen under Einstein's direction. The night before the official reopening, all workers received a telegram from Einstein's dean, directing them to attend a meeting in the Lincoln Hospital auditorium at 8:30 A.M. on Monday before returning to their regular assignments. The dissident workers went to the meeting—only to walk out en masse and throw up picket lines around the hospital itself. Sixty-seven workers taking part in the demonstration were immediately suspended. As the week wore on, the workers continued to man a token picket line, and, because they were under continual harassment in the annex, began setting up alternate services for their patients at a nearby Catholic church which supported their action. The workers made one attempt to reoccupy the hospital-based mental health clinic, but the (city) hospital administrator called out the police to rout the group. In the ensuing melee, twenty-three profession-

als, nonprofessionals and medical students from Albert
Einstein were arrested on charges of criminal trespass.
Even after the arrests, many of the workers held out for
two more weeks. They offered "liberated" mental health
services in the neighborhood church, and called together
regular meetings with community people—including patients who used the Lincoln services, local priests and
nuns, a militant Puerto Rican youth organization, members of the Black Panther Party and representatives of
social service agencies in the Lincoln Hospital area. This
was the first case in which south Bronx residents had been
brought into health policy-making on anything but the
most limited, token advisory basis. In the community
meetings, the discussions ranged over the issues of what
mental health services have meant traditionally, what they
should become, and how community control could bring
about the needed changes. These meetings, some held in
the hospital auditorium and others in local churches or
meeting places, were often highly emotional, but usually
ended with a spirit of unity and common purpose.

Meanwhile, immediately after the walk out, a negotiating team chosen by the workers (including blacks, Puerto
Ricans, whites, professionals, and nonprofessionals) carried the dissidents' demands to the bargaining table, where
they found representatives of the city health agencies, Einstein, and Yeshiva allied against them. The representatives
of Einstein and Yeshiva did not take the negotiations seriously. After three days of half-hearted participation and
amidst behind-the-scenes attempts to play off one group of
workers against another—professional *versus* nonprofessional, black *versus* Puerto Rican—management abruptly
withdrew from the talks and issued an ultimatum to the
workers to immediately accept new assignments. 1199 did

not participate in the abortive negotiations on the ground that the takeover and ensuing strike were violations of the no-strike clause in the union's contract with Einstein. The city's continuing objective, despite the collapse of the talks, was to restore Einstein to the helm at the Lincoln community mental health center with a minimum of fuss. As soon as it became apparent that the Lincoln workers were mobilizing considerable community and outside support, the city Commissioner of Hospitals and Commissioner of Mental Health attempted to enlist their own community support. They called a meeting of the Lincoln Hospital Lay Advisory Board, a heretofore defunct group of businessmen, clergy, etc., who had been appointed as hospital advisors by the city Hospital Commissioner in the mid-fifties. Few of the Board members even lived in the south Bronx; they had not met for over a year. There was every reason to expect that the reassembled Lay Board would unanimously denounce the Lincoln workers. But the Department of Hospitals had misjudged its constituency. Irritated by the Hospital Department's haste in calling the meeting (invitations were telegrammed) and by the clearly one-sided nature of the briefings, a couple of Lay Board members invited representatives of the dissident workers to the meeting. After hearing their story, the Board split; though the Board endorsed the city's position, the motion was passed over several dissenting opinions. Three board members were so moved by the workers' statements that they wrote an open letter to the Governor, the Mayor, and the leading public health officials, which said, in part:

> Community control, real genuine community involvement on the one hand, and the Lincoln Hospital Lay Advisory

Board on the other, are entirely different matters. If the LHMHS community, non-professional employees' and professional supporters' fight to stop the criminal abuses and malpractices, and improve life-and-death community services, is to have lasting value, this fight cannot be smothered by Einstein College of Medicine, Yeshiva University, and [Lincoln Hospital Administrator] Dr. Michelin's attempt to use the Lincoln Hospital Lay Advisory Board, as presently constituted, as a tool. . . . [We] support without reservation the LHMHS non-professional and professional staff efforts to make the services more responsive to the community.

Einstein showed a little more skill and imagination in its search for community support than the city health officials had. The medical school went straight to the top of the south Bronx's Puerto Rican power structure, to the one man who controlled virtually all antipoverty funds flowing into the area. They proposed that he help set up a new community advisory board for Lincoln Hospital and its mental health center. The new board would be dominated by representatives from the community poverty programs and selected members of the old Lay Advisory Board. Since many of the Puerto Rican workers at L.H.M.H.S. owed their jobs to the poverty program and its leaders, such a board could have been effectively used to split the black and Puerto Rican workers. This plan was set aside when the Puerto Rican political leader appeared at a large meeting of workers and community people to present his (and Einstein's) plan. Most people at the meeting challenged his advisory board and told him that the days of token representation were over. Until Einstein was willing to concede power, they said they would have nothing to do with such a plan. He was forced, at least on the face of it, to concur and to abandon any fast arrangement with Einstein.

As is often the case with struggles involving low-income community people, the existing power structure is at considerable advantage simply because it can hold out longer. Once Einstein suspended the workers and cut off their paychecks, the fight began to falter. When it was apparent resistance was on the decline, Local 1199 stepped in and took over the negotiations. The terms they reached and agreed to were

"(1) All employees will return to work on April 9, 1969. There is to be no discrimination or change in status in any form against any employee. There are to be no subsequent proceedings in relation to this matter. This shall in no way be interpreted to prejudice the union's insistence on full pay for all employees.

"(2) Yeshiva University will use its good offices to prevail upon the New York City authorities to drop all charges in any pending criminal action involving the employees.

"(3) Both parties will meet at 10:00 A.M. April 11, 1969, to negotiate outstanding grievances." [The "outstanding grievances" referred to all had to do with job security, hours and pay; the demands for a voice in policy were jettisoned.]

The workers' action had challenged the very nature of the mental health services and raised the right of people (workers and community) to control those services which affect their lives. But, in the end, it was reduced by the union to conventional demands over security and pay. Many of the workers, however, as they returned to work under Einstein in early May, felt they had won at least a partial victory. Einstein had dumped Dr. Peck, the mental health center director, had reassigned his two associate directors to positions elsewhere in the Einstein empire, and had verbally promised that a temporary community board would be set up pending elections of a representative body. The workers were also told that they could elect a board to administer the center internally, and that this board and the community board would have a voice in the selection of an interim director for the mental health center. But, within a few weeks after they had returned to work, the workers learned that Einstein had named a new director without consulting either workers or the community. And, as the weeks passed, the workers realized that Einstein had no intention of helping set up a viable, representative community board to control the center.

But Einstein's victory was not unflawed. Somewhere along the line, the medical college realized that it could not afford the risk of another Lincoln mental health center takeover, and it cautiously decided to pull in its horns. Einstein moved to set up a safe and lasting claim on mental health services in the south Bronx—a new Department of Psychiatry for Lincoln Hospital. The Department, a strictly academic venture, will be safely immune from any upheavals in the community. And, as a side effect, the creation of the department will split the mental health workers, some of whom will be assigned to the department inside the hospital, while others will remain in the community mental health center.

In July 1969, a Federal investigation of the center's finances materialized. The findings of the investigating committee confirmed many of the workers' most strident accusations of fiscal ineptness and mismanagement, but the committee's recommendations did little more than endorse the moves which Einstein had already decided to take. The National Institute of Mental Health sponsored committee did not recommend that the mental health center funds go to a more responsible agent than Einstein, perhaps even to a community-worker board, but merely requested that funds for Lincoln Hospital be separated from those for the mental health center. Einstein was happy to comply, since this separation went along with the recent formation of a Lincoln Hospital Department of Psychiatry. Rather than make the fundamental changes in administrative structure that were indicated, the feds thus merely slapped the wrists of the Einstein emperors—and directed the mental health center to get itself in shape or dismantle.

XIX

THE COMMUNITY REVOLT:

RISING UP ANGRY

There was something for everybody in the Great Society's cornucopia of health programs: Regional Medical Programs for the victims of heart disease, cancer, and stroke; Medicare for the aged; Medicaid for the poor; and neighborhood health centers for the poorest—the urban ghetto-dwellers. Neighborhood health centers, more than any other program, carried the weight of liberal hopes for a fair and rational health system. To Washington health planners, they represented "a totally new approach to the delivery of health services for the poor." The new health centers, financed by the Public Health Service or the Office of Economic Opportunity (O.E.O.), would be everything that hospital outpatient departments are not. Instead of providing care which was fragmented along the lines of medical specialities, they would provide comprehensive general care, oriented towards the whole person, and the whole family. One of the models which most influenced the neighborhood health centers designers was New York City's Gouverneur health center, which had been providing comprehensive outpatient care to residents of Manhattan's lower east side since the early sixties. If it worked at Gouverneur, why not try it in Watts, in Cleveland, and in Philadelphia?

Today, neighborhood health centers are far less popular in Washington, or even in local city halls. "All in all," said one New York government health planner, "they probably caused more trouble than any riots they were supposed to head off." No sooner were they off the drawing boards than neighborhood health centers became the battlegrounds for the first major confrontations between urban medical empires and urban ghetto communities. They were, as some analysts are beginning to understand retrospectively, almost set up for this kind of conflict. Federal regulations called for formal community participation in health center operation, and at the same time stipulated that the centers be affiliated with a qualified back-up hospital. Somehow, in the setting of a new center, community representatives were supposed to be able to participate in a common venture with the men who ran the local medical center, with its hated wards and clinics. Somehow, the medical center representatives were supposed to suddenly show respect for the judgment of the people they had formerly seen only as teaching material. In Los Angeles, Denver, Boston, and a host of other cities, neighborhood health centers have been torn by the conflict between community needs and medical empire priorities.

New York City's Gouverneur, the early model neighborhood health center, has been the scene of one of the nation's bitterest community-medical center conflicts. The lower east side, the community served by Gouverneur, is not a typical urban ghetto, but it is certainly the nation's archetypical ghetto. First the lower east side was an Irish and Italian slum, then a Jewish ghetto, and now increasingly a Puerto Rican and black ghetto. Residues of all the past waves of immigration have remained to create the present mix of Puerto Ricans, blacks, Russians Jews, Polish Catholics, and even Chinese. Despite this diversity, the lower east side is probably the most highly organized ghetto in the country, with a maze of ethnic clubs, political organizations, and special interest groups spanning all ethnic groups and political tendencies. Medically, the region is equally well-organized, with all resources centered around one of the two major medical centers: the New York University Medical Center and the smaller Beth Israel Medical Center. The lower east side's municipally owned health facilities are divided between the two. N.Y.U. runs Bellevue Hospital, and Beth Israel runs the Gouverneur health center.

The history of lower east side community action on health issues goes back to the time, more than a decade ago, when Gouverneur was a city hospital, not a health center. By the late fifties, the old Gouverneur hospital had deteriorated beyond repair. Faced with community demands that it not be closed down entirely, the city made plans to build a new general care hospital, while using the old building as a clinic. In 1961 Beth Israel signed a contract with the city to operate the Gouverneur clinic, or health center, and in 1963, the ground was broken for the new Gouverneur hospital. Construction was three years underway when the Health and Hospital Planning Council (see chapter XIV) announced that the lower east side already had enough hospitals—the new Gouverneur would have to be built as a chronic care home for the aged. The reasons for this mandate were (1) the development of new middle-income housing in the lower east side, which would mean that the demand for municipal hospital care would gradually decline, (2) the existence of five other general hospitals in the lower east side, and (3) a decline in the occupancy rates (the percentage of beds filled at a given time) of the lower east side's hospitals in the early 1960s. Following the Health and Hospital Planning Council's directive, the City suspended construction of the new Gouverneur Hospital, in order to revise its architectural plans. The community responded with a single, angry voice. Old people, the supposed beneficiaries of the proposed chronic care home, insisted that they wanted a real hospital, not a nursing home. Young families in the Gouverneur area pointed out that the five lower east side hospitals were all at least two bus rides away from their homes —a long trip for pediatric or maternity care. A loose, multi-racial community coalition formed around the hospital issue, and in 1966 collected 10,000 signatures on a petition demanding that the hospital be built as a general care institution. Community people began to question all the experts' arguments: Why couldn't the new middle-income families use a municipal facility too? Why such a concern for hospital bed occupancy rates when people knew how hard it was to find a bed even in an emergency? (Occupancy rates in the lower east side's voluntary hospitals climbed to about ninety-one percent in 1968, although eighty to eighty-five percent is considered the maximum rate consistent with safety.) No answers came forth from the city or the planning council, and the community health coalition escalated its struggle with more petitions and demonstrations. In January 1967, the city proposed a compromise: the new Gouverneur hospital would have 120 general care beds and eighty-five chronic care beds, but no maternity or surgical services. It was a victory for the community, but a partial one.

The struggle over the Gouverneur hospital produced the line-up of forces which collided months later in the Gouverneur health center—Dr. Ray Trussell, director of Beth Israel, on the one hand and the Lower East Side Neighborhood Health Council-South on the other. Dr. Ray Trussell, in his former post as the City Commissioner of Hospitals, headed the commission that had originally recommended that the old Gouverneur hospital be closed; just as the hospital closed, Dr. Trussell signed, as hospitals commissioner, the contract which assigned Beth Israel to run the old Gouverneur as an outpatient clinic. Trussell had great influence on the Health and Hospital Planning Council, which subsequently decided to block a new Gouverneur general care hospital. A few years later, Dr. Trussell, no longer Hospitals Commissioner, left his post at Columbia Medical Center to become the dirrector of Beth Israel. (See chapter IV for more on Trussell's influence in New York City health politics.) Meanwhile, the community group which had spearheaded the drive for a new Gouverneur general care hospital had taken permanent form as the Lower East Side Neighborhood Health Council-South (L.E.S.N.H.C.-S.). In 1967, when Beth Israel applied for O.E.O. funds to supplement city support of the Gouverneur health center, L.E.S.N.H.C.-S. was the strongest community health organization on the scene. To comply with O.E.O. requirements for community participation, Beth Israel was forced to accept L.E.S.N.H.C.-S. as the official community board for the Gouverneur health center.

No sooner was L.E.S.N.H.C.-S. ensconced as the official Gouverneur community advisory body than it discovered it had no real voice in the health center's operation. The health center, though certainly far more pleasant and popular than the clinics at Bellevue or Beth Israel, had shown little interest in street-level, preventive health measures. The community, on the other hand, was concerned chiefly with the diseases whose victims usually never arrived at the health center—diseases like narcotics addiction and lead poisoning. Lead poisoning, because of its insidious development and disastrous consequences, is a constant worry for parents in ghetto neighborhoods. Tenement walls are often covered with cheap lead-based paint. The paint peels off as the buildings age, and falls into the hands of little children, who often manage to eat it. Two things can happen to the child who has eaten lead paint. He may become severely and visibly ill, with convulsions leading possibly to death. Or, what is worse, he may show no symptoms at all for years, and then turn out to be mentally retarded. The Scientists Committee for Public Information has estimated that there are 30,000 undiscovered cases of lead poisoning in New York City—enough to alarm every tenement-dwelling parent.

Lead poisoning, however, is easy enough to treat once it has been detected, and it is reliably detected by a blood test. The L.E.S.N.H.C.-S. proposed, in late 1968, that Gouverneur health center undertake an active community-wide program to screen for lead poisoning. But when Beth Israel submitted its 1969 O.E.O grant proposal to L.E.S.N.H.C.-S. for review, the health council was surprised to see that no program for lead poisoning detection had been included. Beth Israel explained that it had already conducted a sample screening of one hundred children on the lower east side, and not found a single case of lead poisoning. Ergo, there was no lead poisoning on the lower east side, and Gouverneur did not have to bother looking for it.

The health council couldn't believe it. Everybody in the neighborhood knew of someone whose children had lead poisoning. In a tumultuous meeting with Beth Israel representatives, L.E.S.N.H.C.-S. members shouted, "It's *our* children who are at stake—not yours. You ought to run a lead poisoning program just to convince us that our children aren't in danger!" Retreating to do a little homework on lead poisoning detection, L.E.S.N.H.C.-S. came up with some disturbing new data. First, Beth Israel's study had been conducted in the winter, the season when lead poisoning reaches its lowest ebb. Second, Beth Israel had used a method of evaluating blood lead tests which many experts considered inaccurate. Finally, Beth Israel had not admitted a single child for lead poisoning in over six years, and with that record, the medical center would be reluctant to admit that lead poisoning really was a problem. Yet in the single month of June 1969, Bellevue had admitted four children for acute lead poisoning symptoms. Despite these facts, it took intense pressure from the L.E.S.N.H.C.-S. to finally make Beth Israel concede to run a small lead screening program out of Gouverneur. On its own the medical center was not interested in lead poisoning, therefore the medical center's health center would not go out looking for it.

Insults followed injury. Throughout 1969 Beth Israel made a series of arbitrary personnel changes at Gouverneur, without ever bothering to consult L.E.S.N.H.C.-S. In one case, a Chinese-speaking clerk, who doubled as a translator for Chinese patients, was suddenly and inexplicably transferred to an evening shift, leaving the Chinese patients to shift for themselves. L.E.S.N.H.C.-S. protested the transfer, and, after some tense discussions, the Chinese clerk was reassigned to the day shift. A few months later,

Dr. Trussell himself gave the order to fire a patient advocate who had been hired by the L.E.S.N.H.C.-S. The excuse—a trivial dispute between the patient advocate and another employee—was transparent to L.E.S.N.H.C.-S., which saw the firing as one more move in the Beth Israel-health council struggle. Citing the O.E.O. regulations, L.E.S.N.H.C.-S. proved that the patient advocate was its employee, not Beth Israel's, and had her reinstated. But when it came to a bigger issue, L.E.S.N.H.C.-S. lost. In the fall of 1969, Gouverneur's administrator resigned. Beth Israel's Dr. Trussell quietly sought out and hired a new man for the job without consulting L.E.S.N.H.C.-S. By the time L.E.S.N.H.C.-S. found out about the new appointment, it was already too late to do anything. Trussell's unilateral appointment clearly violated O.E.O. regulations, but O.E.O. refused to intervene on behalf of the health council.

Alone, the health council had no hope of representing the lower east side community in the operation of the Gouverneur health center. The community could not be mobilized over every single issue that pitted L.E.S.N.H.C.-S. against Beth Israel. And both the city, which owned and in part financed Gouverneur, and O.E.O. which also partly financed Gouverneur, were maintaining a hands-off policy on the Beth Israel health council encounters. But in late 1969 a new force appeared on the scene. A group of Gouverneur workers, all young, all lower east side residents, came to the health council to offer their support against Beth Israel's arbitrary, dictatorial policies.

The workers who decided to ally themselves with the community had first come together in the fall of 1969, when budget cutbacks led Beth Israel to announce imminent job lay-offs. The union's (Local 1199 of the Drug and Hospital Workers) response was to threaten any action necessary, even a strike, if any lay-offs took place. Most of the workers went along with the union's line, but a few felt that a strike would be a betrayal of the community which depended on Gouverneur for health services. The dissidents formed a new group which they called the Health Revolutionary Unity Movement (H.R.U.M.) ("unity" referred to the alliance between workers and community residents). In a series of intense meetings throughout the fall, H.R.U.M. hammered out a complete political perspective on health issues, which they wrote up, leaflet-style, as a "ten-point program." It called for community-worker control of health institutions, free health services, increased preventive services and open admissions to medical schools for minority students.

> We believe that it is the human and constitutional right of all people to govern themselves and make decisions about issues that directly affect their lives and in this way achieve freedom. Now, a small minority of vicious, racist, greedy businessmen and politicians, like those that own the American Medical Association, Drug Companies, Universities, control all the vital health services used against our poor Black, Puerto Rican and white working class communities. This will always happen until the majority (the workers and People) take control of these services. . . . We believe that our peoples are kept sick and weak to support the billion dollar health industry whose profits go to the big businessmen and high salaried doctors. Preventive programs must be implemented to stop vicious attacks on the health of the individuals in our community. These programs must keep people well by changing their living and working conditions. . . . We believe trade unions

must be educated to fight for the political rights of all peoples, not just the narrow self-interest represented by small wage increases or special privileges for a few workers.

The ten-point program ended with an uncompromising challenge.

All union, community, workers and students organizations must support all the points of this political program or be seen as an enemy of the poor people of our communities.

L.E.S.N.H.C.-S. had no difficulty subscribing to the ten-point program, and was soon meeting regularly with H.R.U.M. to plan community health programs which could be launched independently of Beth Israel. H.R.U.M. volunteered to set up, in the workers' spare time, two programs which the health council endorsed: a free breakfast program for neighborhood children, and a patient advocacy program, in which H.R.U.M. members would transport patients to and from Gouverneur, translate for them, help them register, and perform other necessary services. Neither program would have required any contribution of funds or personnel from the official Gouverneur health services progran. But this display of worker and community independence was too much for Beth Israel. When H.R.U.M. members tried to meet at Gouverneur to make plans for the breakfast program, they were met, and dispersed, by city police. Dr. Trussell wrote to the chairman of L.E.S.N.H.C.-S. threatening to close Gouverneur "if any group, including the Council, causes any trouble."

The police intervention at Gouverneur, and the continuing presence of armed guards, struck many of the physicians as entirely disproportionate to the provocation. One physician, who had worked at Gouverneur for three years,

expressed his dismay in a letter to the chairman of
L.E.S.N.H.C.-S.:

> In view of the crisis facing Gouverneur, I feel it is important
> for Gouverneur staff to respond openly to the extreme posi-
> tions taken recently by the Beth Israel administration. In the
> past six months, much of the momentum toward the provision
> of comprehensive health care has been lost, and an atmosphere
> of discouragement and divisiveness prevails. It has become
> increasingly difficult to express dissent from administration
> policy.

Within days, the author of the letter was summarily fired
by Beth Israel. No explanation was given, but since the
dissenting physician was allowed to maintain his admitting
privileges at Beth Israel, it was clear that his professional
competence was not in question.

For H.R.U.M. and L.E.S.N.H.C.-S., this incident was
the last straw. In January 1970, 150 community residents,
called together by L.E.S.N.H.C.-S., marched to Beth Israel and demanded to see Dr. Trussell. They were greeted
by a shoulder-to-shoulder police barricade. In the confusion which followed, four people were arrested. Driven
away from Beth Israel, the crowd returned to Gouverneur,
where they sat in at the director's office for an hour, again
without gaining an audience for their demands. The next
day, nine of the H.R.U.M. workers were suspended from
their jobs, and later five were fired—the leadership of
H.R.U.M. With H.R.U.M. temporarily out of the way,
Dr. Trussell turned on L.E.S.N.H.C.-S. Explaining publicly that L.E.S.N.H.C.-S. was "disruptive" and not truly
interested in the health of the community, he announced
plans to assemble his own, more tractable health council.

The Gouverneur story is not over yet. With literally a

century of struggle behind it, the lower east side community is too old and too experienced to be discouraged by one short skirmish. But already the Gouverneur health center story has entered the establishment mythology of the dangers of community involvement. Perhaps they are right. Gouverneur shows clearly the dangers which await any community, which is too deeply committed to health care to leave it to the experts. First there is the danger of trying to work through formal channels of community involvement, and being rebuffed at every turn. Then there is the danger that as soon as the struggle spills outside of the channels which were meant to contain it, no public agencies (in this case O.E.O. and the City of New York) will be willing to intervene. Finally there is the danger that those who are most committed, who have risked most, will be imprisoned, fired, or otherwise removed from the battleground.

But the danger is ultimately greater for the private medical institutions which ignore the needs and resist the demands of the communities they set out to serve. People who once may have been appeased by the judgment of the medical experts have grown less trusting. People who are today clashing with institutional priorities on the battleground of a neighborhood health center outpost, may tomorrow confront the empire at its core institutions.